IMAGES OF MEMORABLE CASES

IMAGES OF MEMORABLE CASES
50 Years at the Bedside

Herbert L. Fred, MD, MACP
Professor, Department of Internal Medicine
Hendrik A. van Dijk
Former Director of Graphic Communications Group

The University of Texas Health Science Center at Houston

Long Tail Press / Rice University Press
Houston

ricepress.rice.edu

Library of Congress Cataloging-in-Publication Data

Fred, Herbert L.
Images of memorable cases : 50 years at the bedside / Herbert L.
Fred, Hendrik A. Van Dijk. — 1st Rice University Press ed.
     p.; cm.
Includes bibliographical references and index.
ISBN 978-0-89263-000-4 (clothbound) — ISBN 978-0-89263-001-
1 (textbook binding) — ISBN 978-0-89263-002-8 (paperbound)
1. Clinical medicine—Case studies. 2. Diagnosis—Case studies.
3. Clinical medicine—Atlases. 4. Clinical medicine—Case
studies. I. Van Dijk, Hendrik A., 1939- II. Title.
[DNLM: 1. Clinical Medicine—Atlases. 2. Clinical Medicine—
Case Reports. 3. Diagnosis, Differential—Atlases. 4. Diagnosis,
Differential—Case Reports. WB 293 F852i 2007]
RC66.F74 2007
616.07'5—dc22

                         2007018586

Printed by QOOP.

This book is published online in Connexions (http://cnx.org):
http://cnx.org/content/col10449/latest/

Photo credits:
Cover and Cases 15, 34, 61, 66, 77, 150, 151 and 154, Ester Fant
Cases 19, 57, 71, 107, 124 and 149, Michael Callaway
Case 3, Patricia Cernoch; Case 35, Luciano Lemos, MD; Case 44, Margaret
Uthman, MD; Case 67, April Ewton, MD; Case 72, Ethan Natelson, MD;
Case 141, Roger Porter, MD; Case 152, Charles Talakkottur, MD.

DEDICATION

To the resurrection and preservation
of bedside medicine

And to the patients
who made this book possible

ACKNOWLEDGMENTS

We thank Sue Robinson and Kimberley Storrs for secretarial help; Thomas R. Cole, PhD, Director, The John P. McGovern, MD, Center for Health, Humanities, and the Human Spirit, The University of Texas Health Science Center at Houston, for financial assistance; Kenneth E. Sack, MD, Professor of Clinical Medicine, University of California, San Francisco, and Ethan Natelson, MD, Associate Professor of Medicine, The University of Texas Health Science Center at Houston, for critically reviewing the manuscript; and our wives, Judy Fred and Yoka van Dijk, for their love and support.

TABLE OF CONTENTS

Preface   3

Cases and Diagnoses   7

Original Publication Sources   163

Index   167

PREFACE

When sophisticated medical technology became available in the 1970s, it established diagnoses with unprecedented speed and accuracy. But it also affected the practice and teaching of medicine, shifting focus from the bedside to the laboratory and giving rise to a laboratory-oriented rather than a patient-oriented mindset. As a result, physicians' bedside skills have steadily deteriorated, and using one's mind and sensory faculties to make diagnoses has become a lost art.

The images assembled here—some rare, many extraordinary, but every one instructive—are, with few exceptions, related to patients I have personally seen during my 53 years (and counting) as a full-time medical educator. They are presented non-thematically and as unknowns (the way patients typically show up in the hospital emergency department, the clinic, or the doctor's office). Thus, readers must draw upon their entire diagnostic armamentarium in each case.

From the material we provide—limited at times to the image alone—informed readers should be able to make or strongly suspect the correct diagnosis. To find out how you fared, simply turn the page. There you will find the answer and a pertinent commentary. We deliberately have kept the commentaries brief, hoping to stimulate self-learning through additional reading.

The challenge is yours. Enjoy the journey.

Herbert L. Fred, MD, MACP

IMAGES OF MEMORABLE CASES

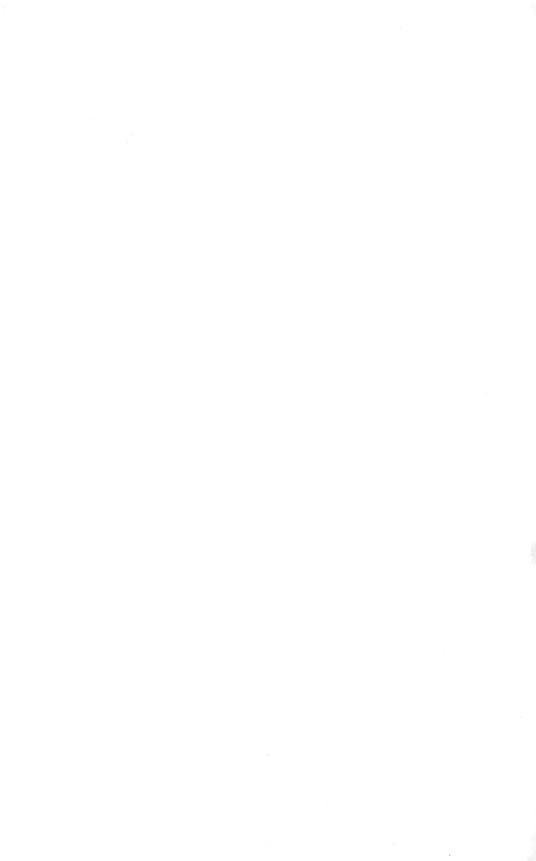

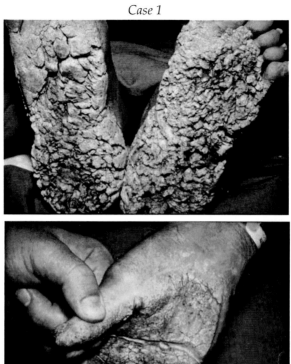
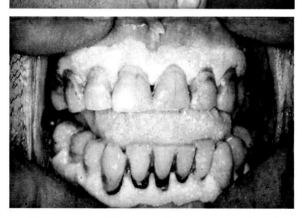

This man could not walk or open his hands
because of the pain induced by the lesions on his
soles and palms. He had no oral complaints.

1. Keratosis palmaris et plantaris. A heredofamilial ectodermal defect transmitted as a mendelian dominant, affecting all races, and appearing in both sexes with about equal frequency. Hyperkeratosis of the palms and soles characterize this disorder, but involvement of the gums and tongue—especially to the extent exhibited by this patient—has not been described heretofore. Moreover the degree of keratosis of his feet (image below) is remarkable, perhaps unique.

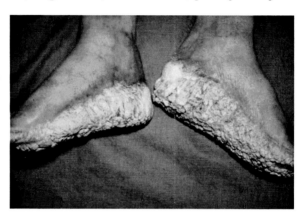

Case 2

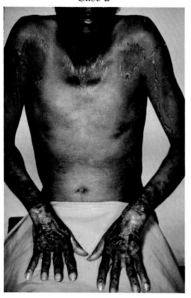

This patient sought medical attention for diarrhea.

Case 3

Peripheral blood film from a man with recurrent fever.

2. Pellagra. Niacin (vitamin B$_3$) deficiency. The dermatologic features of this disorder include desquamation, erythema, scaling, and keratosis of sun-exposed areas, all of which this patient had. Note below the absence of changes in the sun-shielded area.

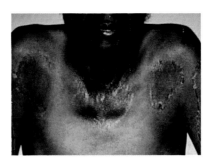

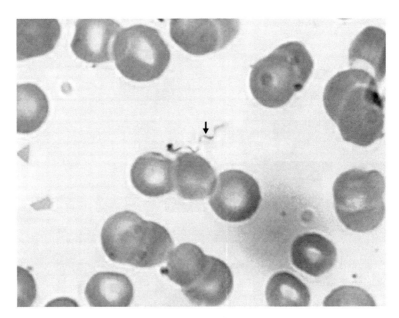

3. Coiled spirochete of *Borrelia hermsii* (arrow). The usual organism causing tick-borne relapsing fever in the United States.

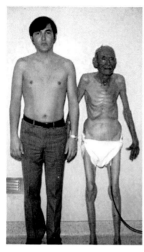 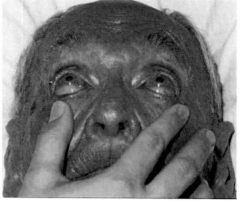

A 92-year-old, asymptomatic Caucasian man.

Case 5

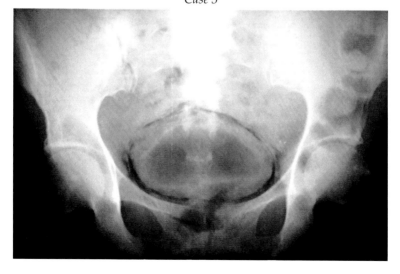

4. Generalized argyria. For many years, this man had used nose drops containing silver. His skin biopsy showed silver deposits in the dermis, confirming the diagnosis of argyria. Although its pigmentary changes are permanent, argyria has no effect on health.

5. Cystitis emphysematosa. Air in the wall and lumen of the urinary bladder. Gas-forming bladder infections typically occur in diabetic patients, and coliform bacteria are the usual pathogens. Urine from this patient, a diabetic, grew *Escherichia coli*. Other organisms, however, such as clostridia, staphylococci, and *Nocardia* and *Candida* species, are sometimes responsible.

Case 6

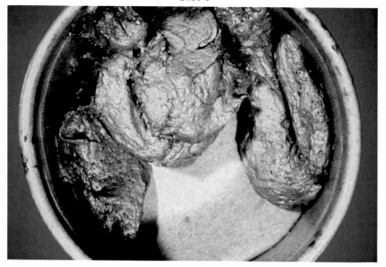

Stool specimen from a patient with epigastric pain, jaundice, and anemia.

Case 7

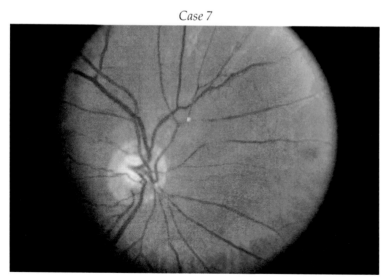

Optic fundus of an asymptomatic 70-year-old diabetic woman.

6. Silver stool. A tarnished-silver or aluminum paint-like stool color characteristically results when biliary obstruction of any type (white stool) combines with gastrointestinal bleeding from any source (black stool). This patient had carcinoma of the ampulla of Vater, the most frequently cited cause of silver stools.

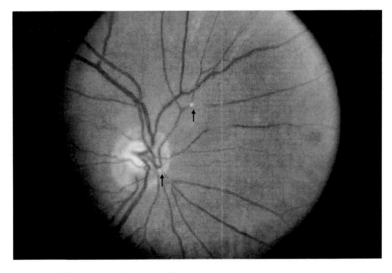

7. Calcific retinal emboli (arrows). These emboli are stark-white, obstruct arteries in or near the optic disk, do not move, and often cause permanent visual impairment. This patient had a calcified mitral annulus, the presumed source of her calcific emboli.

Case 8

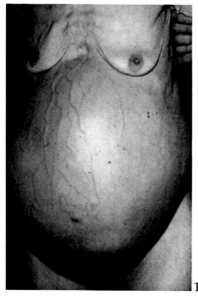

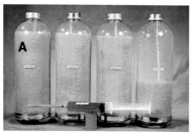

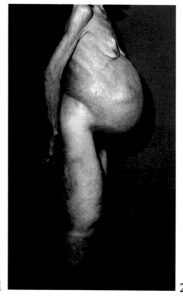

This patient presented with a one-year history of slowly progressive, painless enlargement of her abdomen. She also had Milroy's disease (congenital hereditary lymphedema of the legs). Image 4 shows fluid from paracentesis (A) and a syringe filled with fluid from culdocentesis.

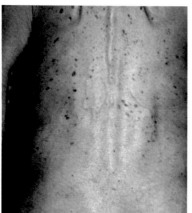

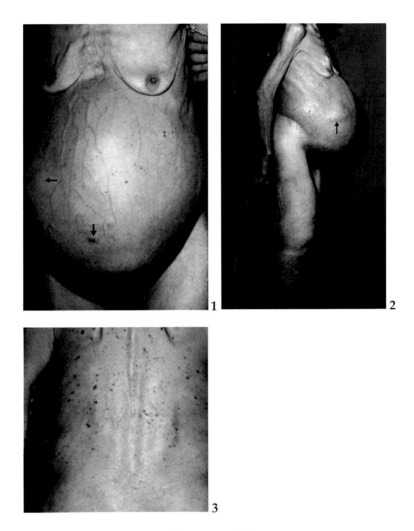

8. Giant cystadenocarcinoma of the ovary (autopsy
proven). Obstructing the inferior vena cava and resulting in
venous collaterals over the abdomen (image 1) and paraspi-
nal area (image 3). Paracentesis yielded gallons of yellowish
tumor fluid (A), while culdocentesis yielded only a small
amount of serosanguineous ascitic fluid. In addition to the
subcutaneous metastases (arrows, images 1 and 2), note the
numerous seborrheic keratoses that had suddenly appeared
on her back—the sign of Leser-Trélat. For more information on
this sign, see Case 129 on page 129.

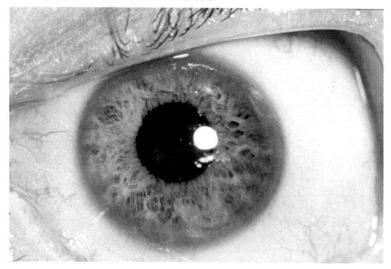

This 32-year-old patient complained of longstanding difficulty speaking. He also had a tremor.

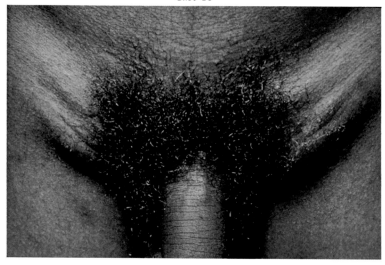

This young adult experienced the acute onset of tender, enlarged lymph nodes in both groins.

9. Kayser-Fleischer ring. Copper deposition in Descemet's membrane of the cornea. These rings can be either dark brown, golden, or reddish-green, are 1 to 3 mm wide, and appear at the corneal limbus. With rare exceptions, they are diagnostic of inherited hepatolenticular degeneration—Wilson's disease.

10. Lymphogranuloma venereum. A sexually transmitted infection caused by *Chlamydia trachomatis*. In this patient, affected lymph nodes above and below the inguinal fold created the "groove sign" bilaterally. Although not pathognomonic, this sign is characteristic of lymphogranuloma venereum and should immediately suggest the diagnosis.

Case 11

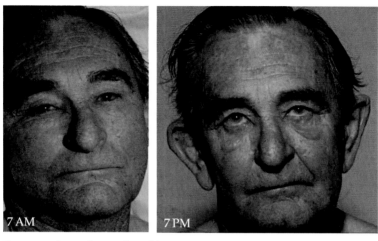

7 AM 7 PM

Same patient. Same day. No treatment.

Case 12

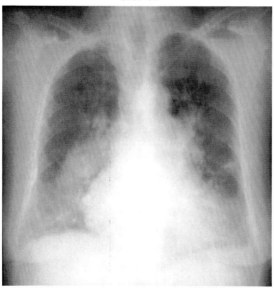

Routine chest radiograph of an asymptomatic 85-year-old woman whose medical history was unremarkable aside from eight uneventful pregnancies.

11. Superior vena caval obstruction. Another diagnostic consideration would be the nephrotic syndrome. In both conditions, facial edema often recedes when the patient remains upright. The patient shown had bronchogenic carcinoma.

12. Atrial septal defect. Secundum type, with left-to-right shunting (proven by transesophageal echocardiography). This is the most common congenital heart disease in adults, affecting women twice as often as men. Without surgical intervention, most of these patients die by age 60. A few, however, do live into their 90s.

Case 13

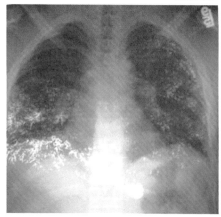 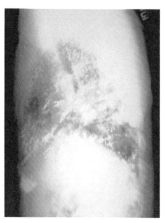

Case 14

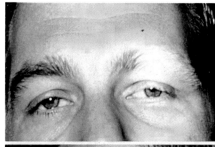

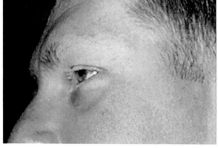

This 27-year-old Hispanic man presented with headache, tinnitus, and blurred vision of several weeks' duration.

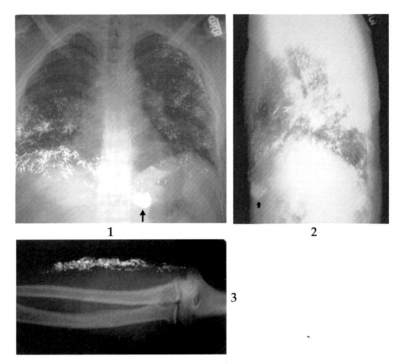

13. Mercury emboli. This patient, a schizophrenic, had injected mercury into his forearm (image 3). Images 1 and 2 show arborizing pulmonary arterioles filled with mercury. Note the pool of mercury in the apex of the right ventricle (arrows).

14. Vogt-Koyanagi-Harada syndrome. The diagnostic clue in this patient is the telltale loss of hair coloring in the left eyebrow and eyelashes (poliosis) with contiguous vitiligo. Additional features of this syndrome—all of which this patient had—include panuveitis, retinal detachment, pinpoint retinal leaks on fluorescein angiography, and evidence of auditory and central nervous system dysfunction, including aseptic meningitis. Decreased visual acuity is the rule. The cause is uncertain, but immune-mediated damage of melanocyte-containing tissue seems likely. Long-term corticosteroid therapy usually halts further ocular damage and often improves vision.

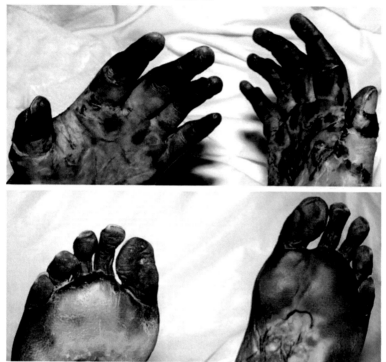

This 47-year-old patient had a one-month history of generalized arthralgias and a two-day history of fever, myalgia, abdominal pain, and diarrhea. His fingers and toes then turned cyanotic and rapidly became necrotic.

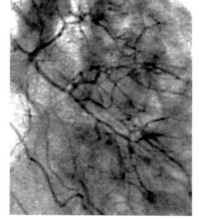

Patient's renal angiogram.

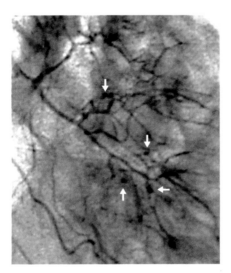

15. Polyarteritis nodosa (autopsy proven). Presenting as symmetric peripheral gangrene. Renal angiogram shows the arterial microaneurysms (arrows) that frequently accompany this disease.

Case 16

This 33-year-old, insulin-dependent diabetic presented with fever, impaired vision, reddish-black nasal discharge, and confusion of two days' duration. He had exophthalmos and external ophthalmoplegia on the right, along with necrosis of the right nasal mucosa and right half of the hard palate. He died 12 hours after admission.

Case 17

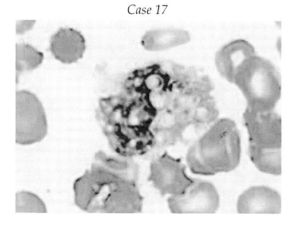

Peripheral blood film from a 40-year-old, terminally ill woman with carcinoma of the cervix.

16. Rhinocerebral mucormycosis. Autopsy demonstrated fungi occluding the right internal carotid artery, severe inflammation of the right orbit, and infarction of the right cerebral hemisphere.

Mucor organisms typically invade and multiply in arteries and veins, leading to vascular occlusion and tissue necrosis. This infection occurs almost exclusively in immunocompromised patients, especially diabetic patients with ketoacidosis.

17. Disseminated histoplasmosis. The leukocyte shown in the blood film contains yeast-phase organisms. Cultures of the blood and bone marrow grew *Histoplasma capsulatum*. Disseminated histoplasmosis typically occurs in immuno-deficient patients, most commonly those with AIDS.

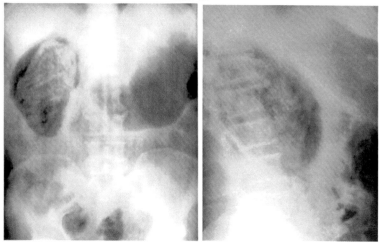

Plain abdominal radiographs of a 72-year-old man with fever, chills, dysuria, and right flank pain. Urinalysis showed proteinuria, pyuria, and gram-negative rods.

Plain abdominal radiograph of an 84-year-old woman who presented with a three-month history of diffuse abdominal pain and weight loss of 40 pounds. On physical examination, she had a hard, nontender, baseball-sized mass in the right upper abdominal quadrant.

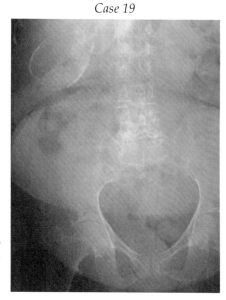

18. Perinephric abscess. In a patient thought to have acute pyelonephritis, the presence of air encircling the kidney is pathognomonic of perinephric abscess. Drainage of this patient's abscess yielded purulent material containing *Proteus mirabilis.*

19. Porcelain gallbladder with probable metastatic carcinoma of the gallbladder. A computed tomographic scan showed that the calcification seen on the plain abdominal radiograph represented the wall of the gallbladder (image below). The scan also showed ascites, multiple lesions in the liver, and nodularity of the peritoneum and small bowel mesentery. These findings suggested metastatic carcinoma of the gallbladder, but the patient refused further investigation.

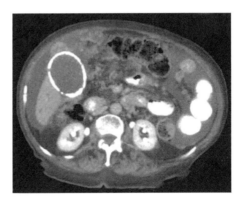

Calcification of the gallbladder wall—referred to as "porcelain gallbladder"— is a rare form of chronic cholecystitis affecting women predominantly. It should always be considered in the differential diagnosis of a calcified lesion in the right upper abdominal quadrant. Confirmation of porcelain gallbladder can be achieved by ultrasonography or computed tomography. Because patients with a calcified gallbladder have an increased risk of gallbladder cancer, cholecystectomy is indicated in most cases.

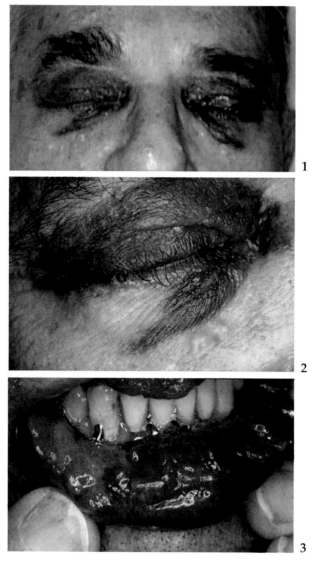

This 60-year-old man said that his eyes turned
black whenever he rubbed them (1). Examination
showed bilateral palpebral hemorrhages and
waxy papules on and near the eyelids (2).
Touching his lower lip with a tongue blade caused
immediate submucosal bleeding (3).

20. Systemic amyloidosis. This patient's "raccoon" eyes, waxy papules on and near the eyelids, and the easily inducible bleeding immediately suggested amyloid disease. Biopsy of a papule showed amyloid in the dermis and in the blood vessel walls.

Case 21

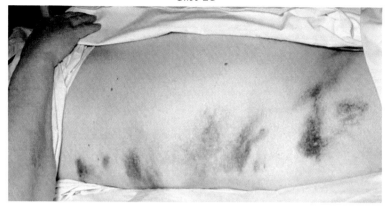

This 40-year-old woman complained of worsening epigastric pain of five days' duration. On examination, she had hypotension, a board-like abdomen, and extensive ecchymoses over her right loin.

Case 22

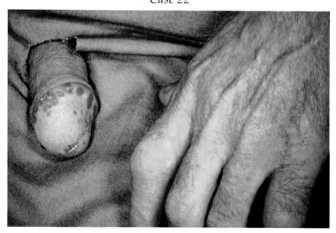

This 27-year-old man complained of pain and swelling in his right knee and left index finger of one month's duration. Three weeks before onset of these complaints, he had had a five-day bout of diarrhea. Shortly before admission, he noticed a pain-less rash on his glans penis.

21. Hemorrhagic pancreatitis. Emergency celiotomy disclosed a boggy pancreas, fat necrosis of the omentum, and reddish-brown peritoneal fluid. The ecchymotic discoloration of her loin—Turner's sign—is not specific for pancreatitis. In the absence of trauma or blood disorders, it is a manifestation of retroperitoneal or intraabdominal hemorrhage.

The image shown displays another indication of retro-peritoneal hemorrhage—ecchymotic patches on the antero-lateral surface of one or both thighs just below the inguinal ligament (Fox's sign). The discoloration (arrows) presumably results from bloody fluid tracking extraperitoneally along the fascia of the psoas and iliacus muscles, becoming subcutaneous in the upper thigh.

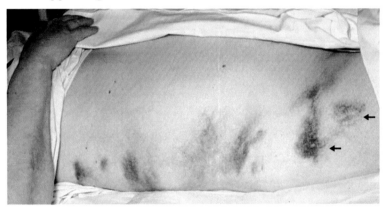

22. Reactive arthritis. Formerly called Reiter's syndrome. The image shows balanitis circinata and fusiform swelling of the proximal interphalangeal joint, both features of this sterile, inflammatory arthropathy. Infections of the urinary tract or gut typically trigger this disorder.

Case 23

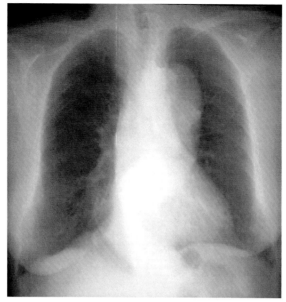

Chest radiograph of an asymptomatic 68-year-old woman whose medical history and physical examination were unremarkable.

Case 24

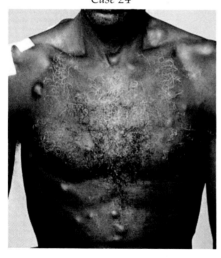

This 51-year-old smoker presented with a three-month history of nonproductive cough and bumps on his skin. The bumps were nontender, firm, and freely movable. Chest radiograph showed a left hilar mass.

23. Chronic aortic dissection. On close inspection, the distance between a calcified plaque in this patient's aortic arch and the outer edge of the arch was 2 cm (normal, <1 cm), suggesting dissection. Contrast-enhanced CT scan of the chest (image below) confirmed the diagnosis by demonstrating a true and false lumen separated by an intimal flap (arrow).

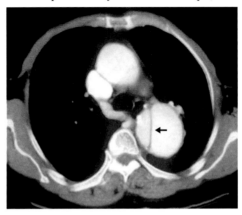

24. Cutaneous metastases from undifferentiated bronchogenic carcinoma. Cutaneous metastases can arise from almost any organ. They usually are papulonodular, painless, discrete, and freely movable. Biopsy is necessary for exact diagnosis.

Case 25

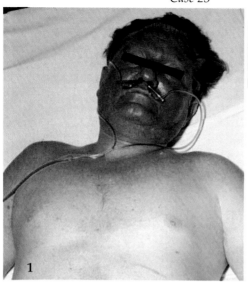

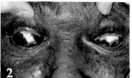

Case 26

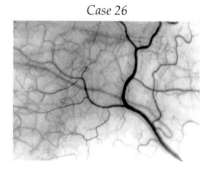

Normal conjunctival circulation (approximately x35).

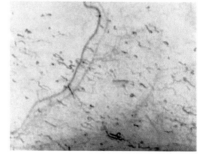

Conjunctiva of a profoundly anemic teenager (approximately x30).

25. Traumatic asphyxia. This condition results from a severe compressive or squeezing injury to the upper abdomen or thorax. The consequent sudden rise in intrathoracic pressure forces a large volume of blood cephalad, causing distention of capillaries and venules in the head and neck. This rapid-fire sequence of events leaves the victim with a never-to-be-forgotten, pathognomonic appearance—striking bluish-red to bluish-black discoloration of the face, neck, and upper part of the thorax (image 1), along with massive subconjunctival hemorrhages. Commonly, these hemorrhages cover only the interpalpebral areas where there is little counterpressure from adjacent tissues (image 2). About 90% of victims who survive for an hour or more will recover, usually completely. *There is no differential diagnosis!*

The patient shown was working in his barn when a bale of hay fell from its mooring and pinned him to the ground. After temporarily losing consciousness, he was able to extricate himself and call for help. He made a full recovery.

26. Sickle cell disease. Inspection of the conjunctiva with the +40 lens of the ordinary ophthalmoscope can be a useful adjunct to the diagnosis of certain types of sickle cell disease, particularly the homozygous form. The characteristic sign consists of sharply defined, dark-red, comma-shaped or cork-screw-shaped vessel fragments that appear isolated from the rest of the conjunctival circulation. These anomalous segments are visible primarily in that part of the lower bulbar conjunctiva covered by the lid.

The pathogenesis of this conjunctival sign remains speculative. There is evidence, however, that endothelial proliferation with trapping of erythrocytes occurs in the distal portion of some capillaries; immediately proximal to such involvement, the vessels are dilated and thin-walled. Infusion of blood or inhalation of oxygen can modify, if not temporarily eliminate, the sign. Conversely, eye drops that contain vasoconstricting agents can render the sign more conspicuous.

Case 27

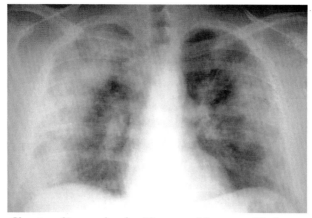

Chest radiograph of a 32-year-old man with fever and nonproductive cough of two weeks' duration.

Cases 28 & 29

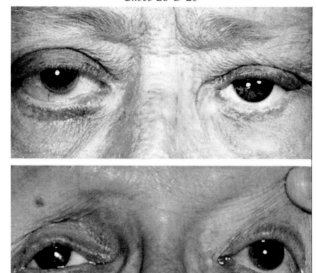

27. Eosinophilic pneumonia. Diffuse infiltrates in the periphery of both lungs, with relative sparing of the perihilar regions, is characteristic of eosinophilic pneumonia. This patient's total leukocyte count was 18,000/mm^3 with 20% eosinophils. After a week of corticosteroid therapy alone, his symptoms, radiographic abnormalities, and eosinophilia resolved.

28 & 29. False eye with hyperbilirubinemia. One patient lost her left eye (top) from trauma and now has pancreatic carcinoma. The other lost her right eye (bottom) from ocular melanoma four years earlier and now has massive hepatic metastases.

Unilateral scleral icterus can appear under two circumstances: 1) the patient is jaundiced from whatever cause, and the nonicteric eye is false, or 2) the serum bilirubin is normal, and the icteric sclera reflects a resolving subconjunctival hemorrhage.

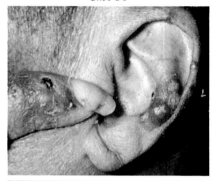

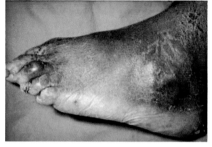

Case 31

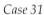

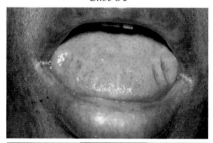

This 53-year-old college professor could no longer lecture because her tongue kept getting in the way. Her tongue was enlarged and had serrations, reflecting imprints of her teeth. Her upper-torso muscles were grossly hypertrophied and hard as wood; they looked like "shoulder pads."

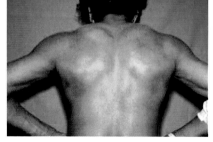

30. Tophaceous gout. The nodules on this patient's finger, ear, toe, and external maleolus are tophi. Diagnostic proof emerged when the tophus on her finger discharged chalky-white material containing needle-shaped sodium urate crystals that were negatively birefringent under polarized light microscopy.

31. Systemic amyloidosis. An enlarged, serrated tongue suggests amyloidosis, acromegaly, or hypothyroidism. The "shoulder pad" sign, however, is relatively specific for amyloid disease. Thus, the combination of an enlarged, serrated tongue with the "shoulder pad" sign is pathognomonic of systemic amyloidosis.

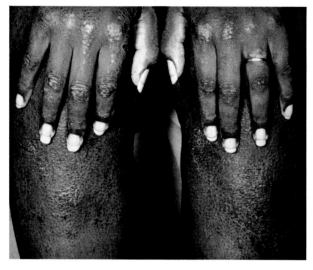

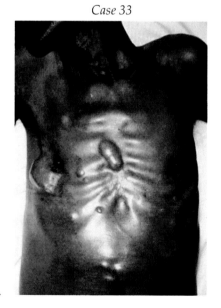

This 56-year-old man sought help for multiple nontender, relatively fixed lesions on his chest and abdomen. The lesion in the right anterior axillary line measured 11 cm in diameter.

32. Dermatomyositis. The erythematous, sometimes scaly, rash of dermatomyositis characteristically occurs on the knuckles of the hands and over the patellae, olecranon processes, and medial malleoli. In fact, violaceous plaques (Gottron's papules) appearing over the metacarpophalangeal and interphalangeal joints—but sparing the dorsal phalangeal surfaces—are virtually pathognomonic of dermatomyositis.

33. Cutaneous metastases from squamous cell carcinoma of the bronchus. This case is noteworthy because the metastases are unusually large.

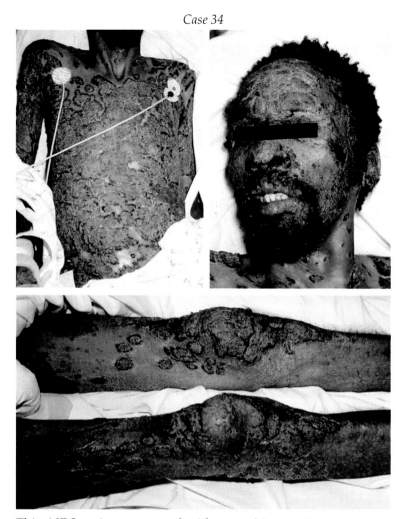

This AIDS patient presented with a pruritic eruption over most of his body. The lesions appeared as sharply demarcated, thick plaques with distinct borders and silvery scales.

34. Hyperkeratotic psoriasis. Biopsies from several plaques established the diagnosis. In patients with AIDS, psoriasis is often severe and refractory to conventional therapy. The differential diagnosis includes Norwegian scabies, mycosis fungoides, and keratoderma blenorrhagica.

Case 35

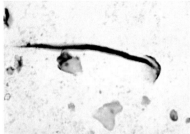

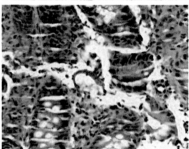

Urine sediment and colonic mucosa from a 53-year-old woman with nonproductive cough, reticulonodular densities on chest radiograph, chronic diarrhea, and recent treatment with large doses of corticosteroids.

Case 36

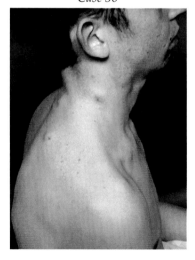

This 12-year-old boy had a long history of bluish, rubbery, nipple-like, cutaneous masses along with recurrent intestinal bleeding.

35. Disseminated strongyloidiasis. The free-swimming worms in this patient's urine proved to be larvae of *Strongyloides stercoralis*. These larvae were also identified in her colonic mucosa (image below, arrows). Although finding larvae in the urine of patients with disseminated strongyloidiasis is rare, it points immediately to the correct diagnosis and prevents what could become a baffling clinical problem with fatal outcome.

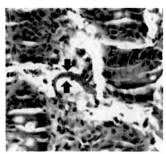

36. Blue rubber-bleb nevus syndrome. A rare, some-times familial, disorder characterized by a variety of cutaneous vascular malformations in association with visceral hemangio-mas. The hemangiomas chiefly affect the gut (image below), are fragile, and bleed easily.

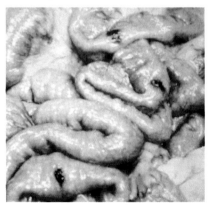

Case 37

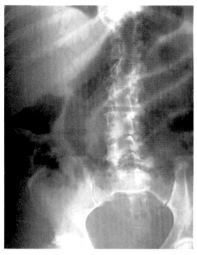

Plain abdominal radiograph of a 60-year-old woman with progressive periumbilical pain and abdominal distention of three days' duration.

Case 38

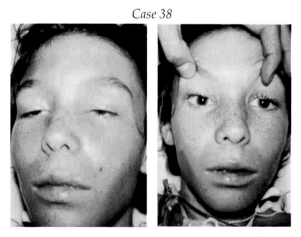

Five days after sustaining a compound fracture of his right arm, this 14-year-old boy noticed that he had blurred vision. Four days later, he could not swallow, move his lips, or protrude his tongue. Other findings included bilateral total ophthalmoplegia with ptosis (left) and dilated, fixed pupils (right). His mental status and sensory examination were normal.

37. Hepatic portal venous gas. The radiographic hallmark of this condition is a spidery pattern of tubular radiolucencies branching toward the liver edge (image below). Gas in the biliary tract is located more centrally and may appear in the gallbladder and extrahepatic biliary ducts as well.

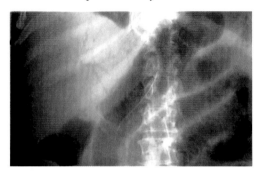

Hepatic portal venous gas usually indicates necrotic bowel in adults and necrotizing enterocolitis in infants. Emergency celiotomy in this patient demonstrated gangrene of the jejunum and gas in the portal vein. Blood cultures grew *Klebsiella* and *Enterococcus* species. The patient died 10 days after surgery.

38. Wound botulism. When symmetric, descending cranial nerve paralysis develops four to 14 days after an open injury and spares mental and sensory function, think of wound botulism. In this patient, culture of serosanguineous fluid from the fracture site grew *Clostridium botulinum*.

Case 39

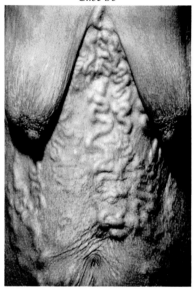

Cases 40, 41 & 42

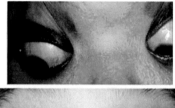

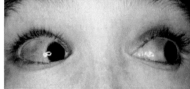

These three unrelated teenaged girls had the same disease.

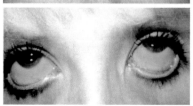

39. Inferior vena caval obstruction. In addition to the gigantic venous collaterals over this patient's abdomen, smaller venous channels (not shown) were visible over the lateral portions of her thorax and along each side of her lumbar spine. The pattern of venous collaterals shown, however, is pathognomonic of inferior vena caval obstruction.

Transfemoral venography in this woman verified total occlusion of her inferior vena cava at its distal end. Although the cause was never identified, she said that her "snakes" had been present for 20 years.

40, 41 & 42. Osteogenesis imperfecta. An autosomal dominant disorder marked by defective formation of collagen. Its cardinal manifestations are blue sclerae, fragile bones, and deafness. The blue discoloration occurs when thinning of the sclera allows the underlying choroid to become visible.

Although blue sclerae occur chiefly in osteogenesis imperfecta, they also appear occasionally in pseudoxanthoma elasticum, Ehlers-Danlos syndrome, and Marfan's disease. Rarely, they are seen in patients with iron deficiency, rheumatoid arthritis, or myasthenia gravis.

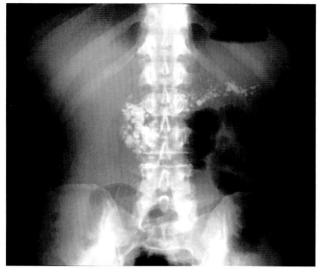

Plain abdominal radiograph of a 44-year-old diabetic with recurrent epigastric pain, nausea, and vomiting. The patient had a long history of alcohol abuse.

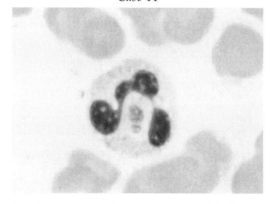

Peripheral blood film from a patient with fever, severe myalgia, thrombocytopenia, and leukopenia.

43. Diffusely calcified pancreas. In this country, alcohol-related pancreatitis is the most frequent cause of pancreatic calcification. The extent of such calcification does not necessarily correlate with the severity or duration of the underlying pancreatitis. Diabetes mellitus is particularly common in these patients.

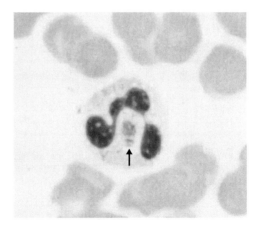

44. Human granulocytic ehrlichiosis. A tick-borne infectious disease caused by *Ehrlichia phagocytophilia*, a small, coccoid bacterium with a Gram-negative cell wall. The leukocyte in the image contains a morula (arrow), a mulberry-like cytoplasmic cluster of ehrlichiae.

Case 45

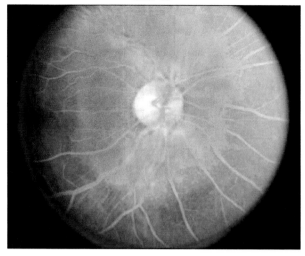

Case 46

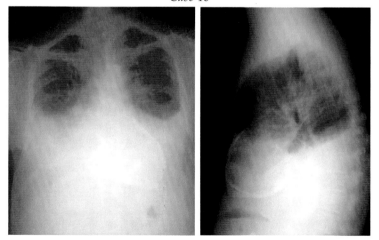

Chest radiographs of a 55-year-old man with distended neck veins, distant heart sounds, hepatomegaly, ascites, and edema of the legs.

45. Lipemia retinalis. As a result of the chylomicron-rich blood within them, all retinal vessels in this disorder appear creamy white, salmon-pink, or yellow-gray. Consequently, arteries are distinguishable from veins only by their smaller caliber. This funduscopic appearance generally occurs only when the serum triglyceride concentration exceeds 4000 mg/dL. In this patient, the serum triglyceride level was 21,040 mg/dL, and the serum looked like cream (image at right).

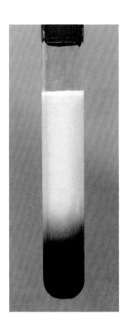

46. Calcified pericardium causing cardiac constriction. The radiographs show striking pericardial calcification. Computed tomography (image below) further delineates the distribution and character of the calcification. The cause of the calcified pericardium in this case is unknown.

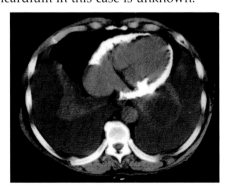

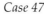

Case 47

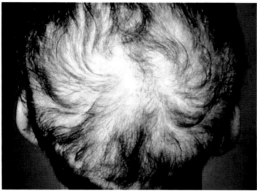

This healthy 16-year-old boy complained that the hair on his scalp had suddenly begun to fall out. Two weeks earlier, he had experienced the abrupt onset of abdominal pain with vomiting, followed several days later by paresthesias in his feet and weakness in his legs. Diffuse alopecia was his only physical abnormality.

Case 48

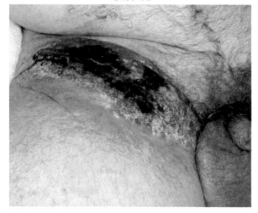

This 27-year-old man complained of fever and increasingly painful "knots" in his right groin. Confident that the patient had infectious lymphadenitis, his physician incised the affected nodes. No pus came forth. The operative site ulcerated, and in a span of two weeks became progressively red, hot, puffy, and tender. Antibiotic therapy had no effect.

47. Acute thallium poisoning. The patient ultimately
admitted that shortly before his symptoms began, he had tried
to commit suicide by swallowing thallium-laden rat poison.
His markedly elevated serum and urine levels of thallium
confirmed his story.

Alopecia is the clinical hallmark of thallium intoxication and
develops in virtually everyone who survives the acute insult.
It usually appears between the first and third week of illness,
characteristically affects the scalp, and commonly spares the
face, axillae, and pubic area. Other manifestations are variable
and nonspecific.

48. Malignant lymphoma, histiocytic type. Biopsy
specimens of a right inguinal lymph node and adjacent
ulcerated skin established the diagnosis. This case has a moral:
When suspecting infectious lymphadenitis, remember
lymphoma.

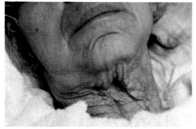

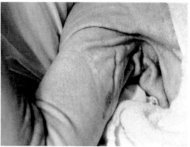

This 42-year-old woman with known angina pectoris experienced black stools and hematemesis of one day's duration. On physical examination, she had greatly diminished femoral, popliteal, and pedal pulses together with angioid streaks in both optic fundi.

Case 50

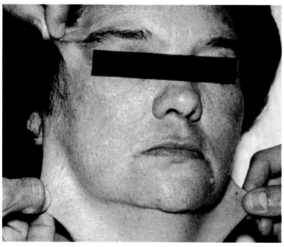

This 40-year-old woman had easy bruisability since child-hood. She also had an inguinal herniorrhaphy as a teenager. An older brother died of massive gastrointestinal hemorrhage.

49. Pseudoxanthoma elasticum. A disorder of connective tissue characterized by degeneration and calcification of elastic fibers in the skin, eyes, and cardiovascular system. The cutaneous changes resemble "plucked chicken skin" and typically appear in the neck and flexural areas. Angioid streaks represent breaks in the elastic lamina of Bruch's membrane beneath the retina. Accelerated atherosclerosis at an early age is common. Gastrointestinal bleeding sometimes heralds the disease and presumably results from altered elastic tissue in the walls of small mucosal arteries.

50. Ehlers-Danlos syndrome.

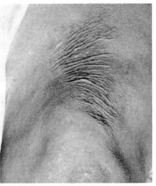

A group of heritable disorders of connective tissue, most of which are autosomal dominant. Characteristic manifestations are easily stretchable skin, spontaneous bleeding, and hypermobile joints. The skin may be soft, thin, and hyperelastic. Scars typically are thin and wrinkly, with a "cigarette paper" quality (top image). Sometimes, however, they appear as small molluscous pseudotumors (bottom image). In some cases, spontaneous arterial rupture occurs and can result in torrential bleeding from the gastrointestinal or urinary tract, tracheobronchial

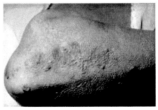

tree, or a gravid uterus. Articular hypermobility sometimes allows extraordinary contortionism.

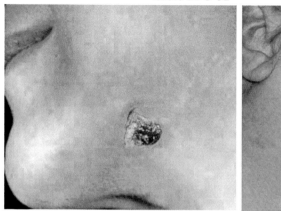 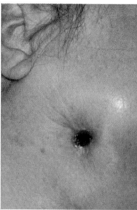

A 42-year-old woman (above left) complained of a painless sore beneath her jaw. The sore had discharged pus intermittently during the previous four years, but numerous trials of antibiotic therapy had been ineffective. A 29-year-old woman (above right) noticed an occasional serosanguineous discharge from a red spot near the angle of her jaw. The drainage was painless and had been present for six months.

Case 53

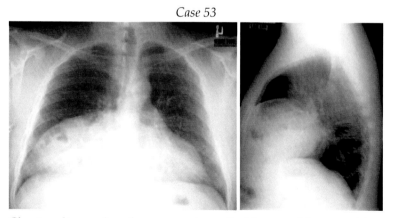

Chest radiographs of an asymptomatic 36-year-old man with normal physical findings.

51 & 52. Dental sinus tract. Dental radiographs in the first patient (left image) showed a periapical abscess of a mandibular molar. After the tooth was extracted, the discharge stopped, and the sore healed. In the other patient, radiographs showed a periapical radiolucency at the root of a maxillary premolar, suggesting pulpal necrosis. Conventional endodontic therapy saved the tooth and cured the discharge.

These two cases illustrate an important clinical point: Most chronically draining sinuses of the face or neck have a dental origin. And because dental symptoms are often absent, diagnosis can be delayed for years.

53. Foramen of Morgagni hernia. The radiographs show that the large, right paracardiac mass represents bowel that has herniated anteriorly into the chest, presumably through a congenital diaphragmatic defect involving the Foramen of Morgagni. A computed tomographic scan (image below) confirmed the diagnosis.

Such herniation typically occurs on the right but can be left-sided or bilateral. Surgical repair is recommended in most cases to prevent obstruction or strangulation of the bowel.

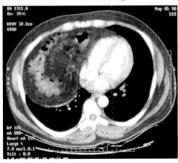

Case 54

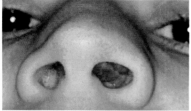

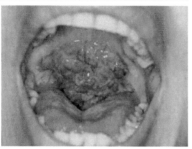

This 14-year-old girl from El Salvador presented with a one-year history of throat discomfort and nasal stuffiness.

Cases 55 & 56

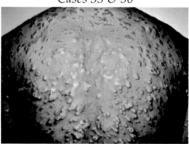

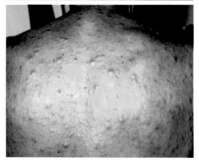

A 23-year-old homosexual man had an intensely pruritic, papulonodular eruption over his arms and back (top image). A 52-year-old man with AIDS had reddish papules and nodules—some pustular—over his face, chest, arms, and back (bottom image).

54. Rhinoscleroma. A chronic, progressive infection of the upper airways caused by *Klebsiella rhinoscleromatis*. Biopsies of the cobblestone-like masses in her oropharynx and left nasal passage showed granulomatous inflammation; culture of the specimens grew the causative organism. Treatment requires surgical debridement and prolonged antibiotic therapy. Most cases occur in developing countries, but because of recent immigration patterns, the incidence of this disease in the United States is increasing.

55 & 56. Secondary syphilis. On dark field examination, the lesions in the homosexual man were teeming with spirochetes. Additionally, his fluorescent treponemal antibody absorption test was positive. The AIDS patient had a penile chancre and a positive serum test for syphilis. With penicillin therapy, the eruption in both patients rapidly resolved.

Dermatologic manifestations are the hallmark of secondary syphilis. Copper-red papules are most common, but macular, pustular, acneiform, psoriasiform, nodular, annular, or follicular variants can appear. The lesions characteristically do not itch, but as shown in the first patient, pruritus can be the dominant clinical feature.

Case 57

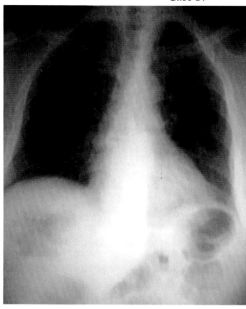

Chest radiograph of a 51-year-old man with fever and shaking chills of two weeks' duration. His physical examination was unremarkable except for a temperature of 104°F.

Cases 58, 59 & 60

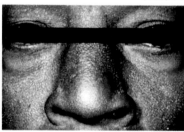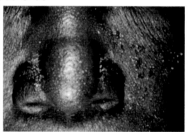

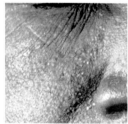

These three patients had the same disease.

57. Pyogenic liver abscess. The chest radiograph shows a peculiar pattern of mottled gas and an air-fluid level in the region of the liver. On computed tomograhic (CT) study of the abdomen, the scout film (below left) shows the gas to be similar in appearance to, but separate from, intestinal gas. The CT scan demonstrates a large liver abscess with an air-fluid level (below right). Drainage of the abscess yielded 600 cc of pus, which grew *Klebsiella pneumoniae*.

This case illustrates the value of the chest radiograph in diagnosing disease *below* the diaphragm.

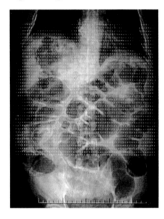 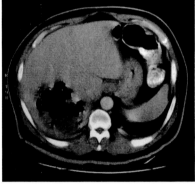

58, 59 & 60. Pellagra. All three images show numerous plugs of inspissated sebum projecting from dilated orifices of sebaceous glands. "Dyssebacia"—the name coined to describe this finding—appears in about one-fifth of pellagrins and constitutes a fifth D of pellagra. The other four are dermatitis, diarrhea, dementia, and death.

On palpation, these plugs feel like sharkskin or sandpaper. They first appear on the alae nasi, then spread over the nose, and in advanced cases involve the forehead, lips, and chin. With niacin therapy, the sebaceous plugs fall out within several days, and the lesions clear completely within a week or so.

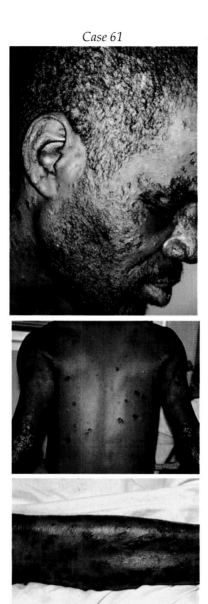

This 42-year-old man had longstanding papules, nodules, and plaques on his face and neck; plaques and psoriasiform lesions on his back, elbows, and axillae; and ichthyotic patches on his legs. All of these abnormalities were asymptomatic.

61. Cutaneous sarcoidosis. Asymptomatic nodules, papules, and plaques on the face, shoulders, or extremities strongly suggest sarcoidosis. Diagnostic confirmation requires histologic demonstration of noncaseating granulomas, negative stains and cultures of biopsy specimens for acid-fast bacilli and fungi, and clinical findings consistent with those of sarcoidosis. The patient shown met all of these requirements.

Case 62

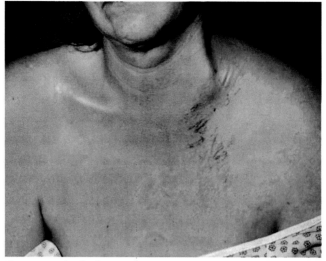

Two months before admission, this 37-year-old woman noticed bluish-red streaks in the skin near her left sternoclavicular joint. Soon thereafter, hoarseness and hemoptysis developed.

Case 63

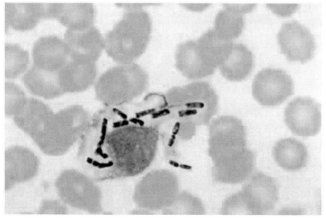

Peripheral blood film from a woman with AIDS who had a two-day history of high fever and shaking chills.

62. Venous stars heralding carcinoma of the lung.

The image shows fullness in the left supraclavicular space; a distended, left-sided, neck vein; striking venous stars (cutaneous venules); and deeper dilated veins in the left upper thoracic area. Biopsy of a hard, left-sided, supraclavicular mass disclosed poorly differentiated squamous carcinoma.

As this case demonstrates, the sudden appearance of venous stars on the upper chest or shoulder may be the earliest manifestation of an obstructed great thoracic vein. Indeed, further study of this patient disclosed total occlusion of her left subclavian and innominate veins. For more information on venous stars, see Case 146 on page 147.

63. Diplococci heralding bacteremia. Blood cultures in this patient grew *Streptococcus pneumoniae.*

The automated blood counters in widespread use today cannot detect pathogens in the peripheral blood film, but the human eye can. Discovering pathogens in the peripheral blood film enables the examiner to make a specific diagnosis on the spot— before results of blood cultures, serologic studies, or other tests become available. Moreover, it allows prompt administration of potentially life-saving therapy. And, as this patient exemplifies, it raises the possibility of an altered immune status, such as AIDS, acquired hyposplenism, hypogammaglobulinemia, or deficiency of certain components of the complement system.

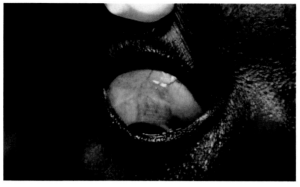

This 41-year-old woman complained of a scratchy sensation in her right eye of three months' duration. On external inspection, her eyes appeared normal, but raising the right upper lid unveiled a salmon-colored conjunctival mass. Physical examination was otherwise unremarkable, and results of conventional laboratory studies were normal.

Case 65

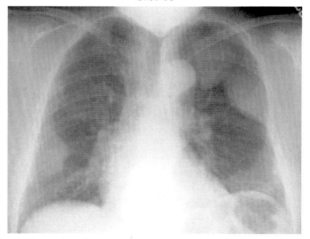

Chest radiograph of a 68-year-old man with a serum calcium of 13.5 mg/dL and a serum electrophoresis showing a monoclonal spike of 4.4 gm/dL. His physical examination, complete blood count, and urinalysis were normal.

64. Conjunctival lymphoma. Biopsy of the mass showed diffuse, well differentiated, B-cell lymphocytic lymphoma. With localized radiotherapy, the conjunctival lesion disappeared.

65. Multiple myeloma. Each of the large masses on the chest radiograph was contiguous with a partially destroyed rib (image below, arrowheads). Biopsies of one of the masses and of the bone marrow showed sheets of plasma cells. The masses, therefore, represented expanding plasmacytomas of ribs rather than pulmonary parenchymal lesions.

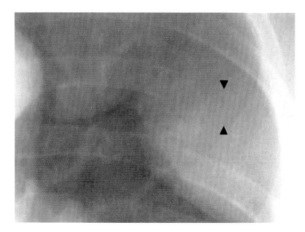

Chest disease in multiple myeloma can manifest as infection or bone lesions, complicated at times by pleural effusion.

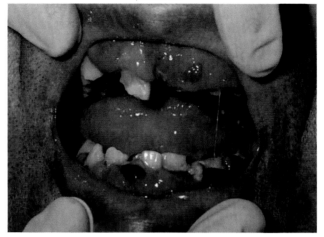

This 55-year-old man presented with a three-week history of diffusely swollen gums that had made eating difficult. On examination, he also had shotty generalized lymphadenopathy, a palpable spleen, and ecchymoses over both legs.

Case 67

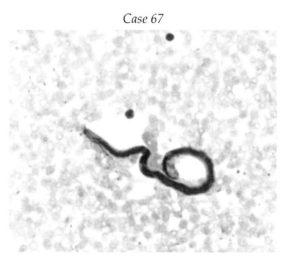

Peripheral blood film from a native of West Africa.

66. Acute myelomonocytic leukemia. This patient's total leukocyte count was 96.2 x 10,000 mm^3 with 12% lymphocytes, 38% monocytes, and 50% blasts. His bone marrow study confirmed the diagnosis.

Major infiltration of the gums by leukemic cells is common in acute myelomonocytic or monocytic leukemia and may be the presenting manifestation. This feature is less frequent in other types of acute leukemia.

Noticeable gingival hypertrophy may also result from several drugs (phenytoin, cyclosporine, nifedipine, diltiazem, verapamil and penicillamine) and from various maladies (scurvy, sarcoidosis, Crohn's disease, amyloidosis, lymphoma, Kaposi's sarcoma, cytomegalovirus infection, Wegener's granulomatosis, and hereditary gingival fibromatosis).

67. Loiasis. The image shows a sheathed microfilaria of *Loa loa*, a threadlike worm distributed irregularly in West and Central Africa. Flies of the genus Chrysops are the intermediate hosts and vectors. Adult worms inhabit the subcutaneous connective tissues of the body, causing localized edema called "Calabar swellings." Occasionally, the adult worm can be seen crossing the eye beneath the conjunctiva. The immature forms (microfilariae) are diurnal and appear in greatest concentrations in daytime blood. Finding the microfilariae in routine blood films establishes the diagnosis.

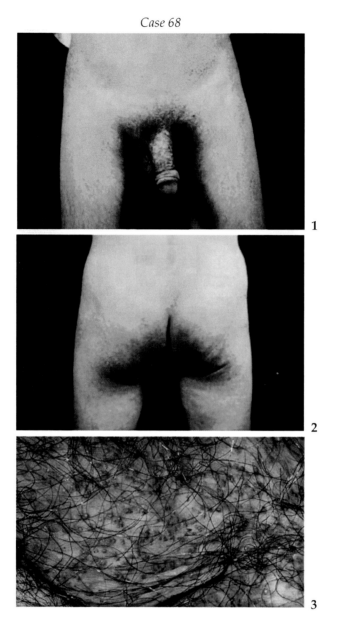

1

2

3

This 38-year-old man suffered for many years from episodes of excruciating leg pains and intermittent tingling sensations in his fingers. His older brother and maternal uncle had died of kidney disease.

68. Fabry's disease (angiokeratoma corporis diffusum). An inborn error of glycosphingolipid catabolism resulting from deficiency of the enzyme α-galactosidase A. Transmitted by an X-linked recessive gene, the enzymatic defect causes widespread deposition of glycosphingolipids, mainly ceramide trihexoside. Affected vessels become narrowed, and the consequent tissue ischemia presumably accounts for many of the clinical features. Women usually are carriers.

The telltale sign of Fabry's disease is the angiokeratoma — distended capillaries protruding into a hyperkeratotic epidermis (image 3). These lesions appear as discrete, punctuate, purple-red papules predominantly in the "bathing suit" area (images 1 & 2).

Another hallmark is pain, often debilitating, and usually in the extremities. It may be constant or may occur in crises that last from minutes to several days.

Additional manifestations include acroparesthesias, cardiac abnormalities, and intracranial events. Renal failure is the usual cause of death.

Prevention is the most effective therapy; hence, genetic counseling is essential.

Case 69

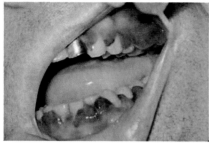

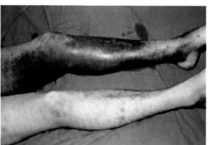

This 30-year-old homeless man had swollen, erythematous gums (top), scattered perifollicular hemorrhages, and extensive ecchymoses over his left leg (bottom). His hematocrit value was low, but his platelet and leukocyte values were normal.

Case 70

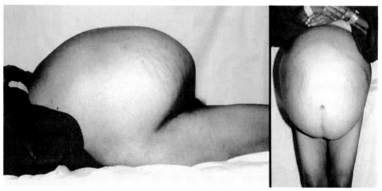

This 49-year-old woman presented with slowly progressive, asymptomatic abdominal swelling of one year's duration. Six years earlier, she had undergone resection of a retroperitoneal liposarcoma. On examination, her abdomen was incredibly enlarged, rock-hard, and nontender.

69. Scurvy. The triad of perifollicular hemorrhages, extensive ecchymoses, and hypertrophied, discolored gums is diagnostic of scurvy. This patient's plasma and leukocyte ascorbic acid concentrations were low. With proper diet and Vitamin C supplementation, his anemia and abnormal physical findings promptly resolved.

70. Metastatic liposarcoma. Computed tomography showed numerous, non-homogeneous masses of varying density compressing and displacing but not invading contiguous abdominal and retroperitoneal organs (image below). At celiotomy, most of the neoplastic tissue was removed in three large blocks totaling 100 lbs! The histopathologic diagnosis was well-differentiated liposarcoma. Patients with this cell type can have a five-year survival rate as high as 80%, while in those with poorly differentiated lesions, survival drops to 20% or less. This patient survived for a total of nine years, ultimately succumbing to widespread metastases.

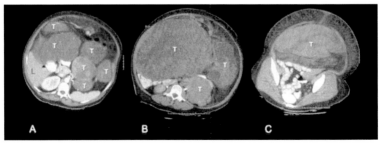

Computed tomography at level of liver (A), mid-abdomen (B), and pelvis (C) after intravenous injection of contrast material. L=liver, T=tumor.

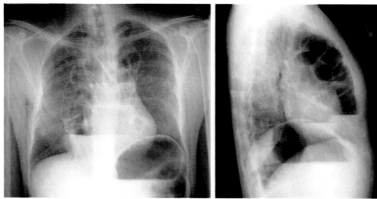

Chest radiographs of a 31-year-old medical resident with recurrent bouts of hiccupping, associated at times with mild epigastric distress.

Case 72

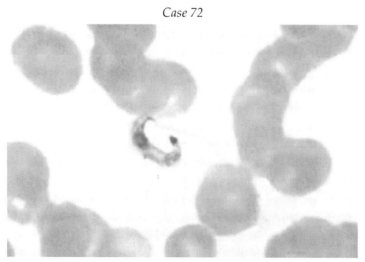

Peripheral blood film from a 10-year-old Brazilian boy with Romaña's sign-- painless, unilateral, palpebral edema with conjunctivitis and swelling of regional lymph nodes.

71. Colon interposition. The chest radiographs show a gas-distended, lobulated, cystic structure with several air-fluid levels, filling the precordial space from the diaphragm to the thoracic inlet. In addition, the lateral aspects of three upper ribs on the right are deformed. These findings together are diagnostic of a segment of colon surgically placed in the chest. A barium swallow shows the intrathoracic segment of colon with a few diverticula (image below).

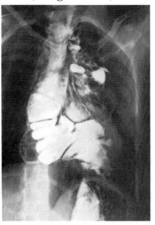

This patient had a congenital tracheoesophageal fistula treated at birth with gastrostomy and at age two with colon interposition between her cervical esophagus and her stomach. She has done remarkably well ever since.

72. Acute Chagas disease (American trypanosomiasis). Shown between red blood cells is a trypomastigote of *Trypanosoma cruzi*. This form of the parasite is visible in the blood only during the acute stage of the disease and is diagnostic. Romaña's sign, which often heralds the acute phase, develops when the vector, a reduviid bug, deposits the parasite on or near the conjunctiva.

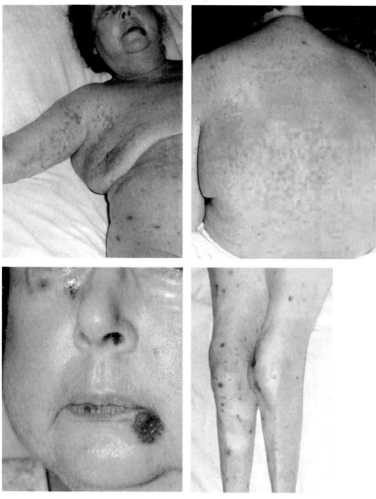

This 65-year-old woman presented with an intensely pruritic, month-long skin rash that started beneath her right breast, then spread quickly to involve multiple sites, including her face. Some of the lesions were maculopapular, others were psoriasiform, and still others were solitary, rounded, and erythematous. She spent six weeks in the hospital undergoing studies before the diagnosis finally emerged.

73. Scabies. A skin biopsy shortly after admission showed nonspecific findings. A repeat biopsy five weeks later uncovered numerous *Sarcoptes scabiei* mites. After several courses of scabicidal therapy, the rash resolved. But the story didn't end there.

Thirty-five hospital workers acquired scabies from this patient. The incubation period for those virgin cases ranged from five to 11 days, a distinctly shorter time frame than the 10 days to a month or more cited in textbooks. Many other personnel who came in contact with this patient never got the disease, including her personal physician who examined her twice daily. A consultant, however, who had had scabies as a medical student, acquired it from this patient and became symptomatic 24 hours after examining her.

Observations in this case teach several lessons: 1) in some patients, diagnosing scabies requires more than one attempt; 2) susceptibility to scabies varies considerably; 3) the incubation period for virgin cases can be much shorter than what the textbooks cite; 4) in cases of repeat infection, the incubation period is only 24 to 72 hours; and 5) any unexplained, persistent, intensely pruritic skin rash should be considered as scabies until proved otherwise.

Case 74

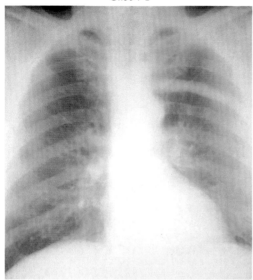

Routine chest radiograph of an asymptomatic 50-year-old man. The same study five years earlier had shown no abnormality.

Case 75

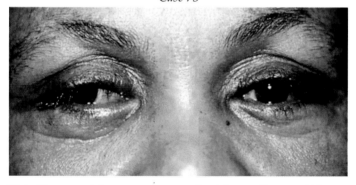

This 51-year-old nurse presented with swollen eyelids, excessive tearing, and photophobia of 18 months' duration. During that time, she had consulted with two internists and four ophthalmologists before the diagnosis ultimately emerged. Topical corticosteroid preparations and other symptomatic treatment had afforded no relief. Except for her eyes, she felt perfectly fine.

74. Metastatic carcinoma of the prostate. The radiograph shows a solitary "white" fourth rib on the left side. Such a finding in a middle-aged or older man should always suggest osteoblastic metastasis, particularly from carcinoma of the prostate. In this patient, biopsies of the prostate and affected rib disclosed adenocarcinoma.

75. Infiltrating lobular carcinoma of the breast metastatic to the eyelids. The mystery in this case began to clear when a CT scan of the pelvis showed osteolytic and osteoblastic lesions. All previous studies, including blood counts, chest radiograph, bone scan, mammograms, and CT scans of the head and orbits, had given normal results. At this time, a thorough physical examination disclosed several cutaneous nodules, 0.5 to 1 cm in diameter, on the patient's upper torso. Biopsy specimens from one of these nodules and from the right lower eyelid showed identical findings: metastatic infiltrating lobular carcinoma of the breast.

Symmetric thickening and induration of the eyelids, presumably from lymphatic obstruction by tumor cells, is a rare form of lid metastases, occurring almost exclusively in women with breast carcinoma. Accordingly, the patient received methotrexate, cyclophosphamide, and 5-fluorouracil. Within two months, her skin nodules had regressed substantially, and her eyelids had returned to normal.

Case 76

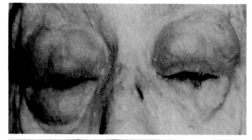

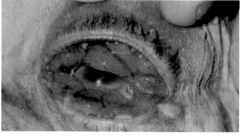

This 84-year-old woman presented with a four-month history of painless swelling of all four eyelids (top). On examination, the lids felt boggy, and each eye had pinkish-pale, lobular tissue covering almost the entire bulbar and palpebral conjunctiva (bottom). Generalized lymphadenopathy and mild normocytic, normochromic anemia were additional findings.

Case 77

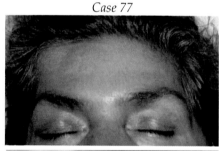

This 62-year-old woman presented with diffuse, debilitating skeletal pain and a 2x3x4 cm painless, firm nodule on her forehead. She also had several smaller nodules of similar nature on her scalp. All of these lesions pulsated.

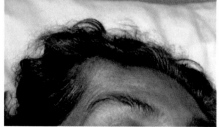

76. Conjunctival lymphoma. Biopsy of a cervical lymph node showed diffuse, small-cell lymphocytic lymphoma. With conventional chemotherapy, the ocular abnormalities improved substantially, and the generalized adenopathy and anemia resolved.

Conjunctival lymphoma usually occurs in persons older than 50 years and affects men and women equally. It can be unilateral or bilateral, with or without systemic involvement. The lesions typically are painless. Definitive diagnosis requires histologic examination and immunohistochemical stains of the involved tissue. Treatment consists of radiotherapy for localized disease and chemotherapy for systemic disease.

77. Metastatic renal cell carcinoma. The primary tumor arose in the left kidney and quickly spread throughout the skeletal system.

As this case illustrates, pulsatile metastases characteristically involve adjacent bones (images below). The point to remember, however, is this: If a metastasis pulsates, the primary tumor is carcinoma of the kidney or thyroid gland. There are no other considerations, unless the sternum is the site of a pulsating metastasis. In that instance alone, multiple myeloma is another diagnostic possibility.

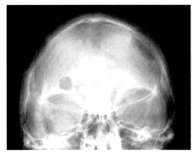 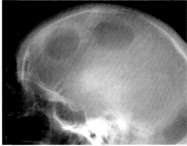

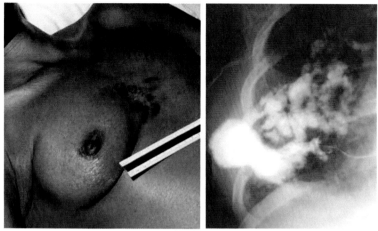

This 50-year-old woman presented with a one-year history of dyspnea on exertion and a two-week history of a painful, swollen right breast. On examination, she had a tender, warm right breast and several draining sinuses in and near her sternum (left image). Chest radiograph showed miliary lesions throughout both lungs. Contrast material injected into a sinus opening demonstrated irregular tracts and cavities in the right breast and chest wall (right image).

Case 79

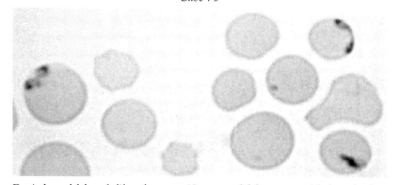

Peripheral blood film from a 60-year-old hunter with headache, malaise, anorexia, and low-grade fever of two weeks' duration.

78. Actinomycosis of the right breast, chest wall, and lungs. The clinical findings suggested tuberculosis versus actinomycosis. Incision and drainage of the right breast abscess showed pockets of pus, but acid fast and fungal stains were negative and cultures grew no organisms. Open lung biopsy, however, showed microabscesses containing sulfur granules. Cultures again were sterile and stains showed no pathogens. Nevertheless, the combination of sulfur granules and draining sinuses pointed strongly to actinomycosis. Accordingly, the patient received high doses of penicillin intravenously for six weeks after which time her sinuses had closed, the breast abscess had healed, and the lung lesions had all but disappeared.

This case may be only the second reported example of miliary lung lesions caused by actinomycosis. It also joins only a handful of reported cases of actinomycotic breast abscess.

79. Babesiosis. The diagnosis of this tick-borne disease depends on finding the causative protozoan in the peripheral blood film. In this patient, the film shows dumbbell-shaped markings in red blood cells, findings characteristic of *Babesia* species (image below, arrows). Not surprisingly, the blood film findings of babesiosis simulate those of *Plasmodium falciparum* malaria.

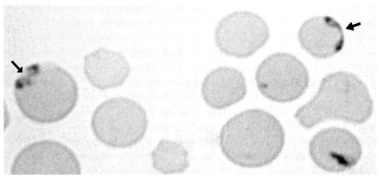

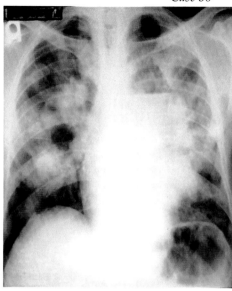

Chest radiograph of a terminally ill 44-year-old man with a five-month history of intermittent fever and cough productive of yellow, blood-tinged sputum. On physical examination, he had a big liver and evidence of substantial weight loss. He died shortly after admission.

Case 81

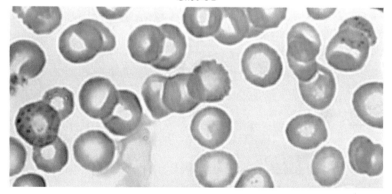

Peripheral blood film from an anemic, 53-year-old geophysicist who complained of fatigue and constipation. The blood film of his asymptomatic wife showed similar changes, but that of his 12-year-old son was normal.

80. Bilateral pulmonary amebiasis. Autopsy disclosed numerous bilateral pulmonary abscesses, up to 15 cm in diameter. The right hepatic lobe also contained a single large abscess that had eroded into the right hepatic vein. The diaphragm was not involved. Countless amebic trophozoites were evident in the walls of the hepatic and pulmonary abscesses. While penetration of a hepatic abscess through the diaphragm is the usual route of amebae to the lungs, this case illustrates that amebae can also reach the lungs by entering the blood stream directly, the diaphragm remaining intact.

81. Lead poisoning. Basophilic stippling of this patient's red cells (image below, arrows) suggested lead poisoning. Despite repeated inquiry, however, no source for such poisoning emerged. The plot thickened when blood lead concentrations were substantially elevated in both the man and his wife but normal in their son. Continued sleuthing ultimately unveiled the culprit — cocktail glasses decorated with lead-based paint. The husband and wife drank from these glasses daily, but their son never drank from them. Washing the glasses by machine presumably caused leaching of lead salts. Chelation therapy for the two adults returned their hematologic findings to normal, and the patient became asymptomatic.

Moral: Basophilic stippling of red cells can be the first, best, or only clue to lead poisoning.

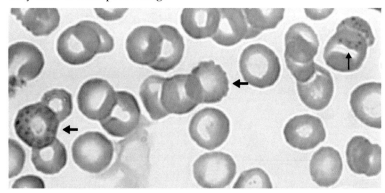

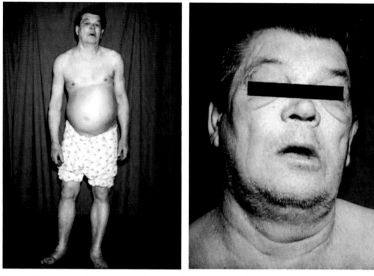

This 57-year-old bartender had longstanding ascites attributed to presumed hepatic cirrhosis.

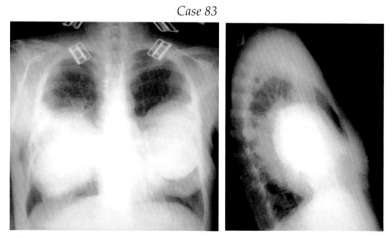

Chest radiographs of a 29-year-old asymptomatic woman with malignant melanoma.

82. Myxedema ascites. Immediate clues to hypothyroidism in this man were his expressionless face, periorbital puffiness, pallor, peripheral edema, and, of course, his massive ascites. Indeed, because it is curable, myxedema should be considered in every patient with conspicuous ascites, except perhaps those with widespread or terminal malignancy. The patient shown received thyroid replacement therapy, and all of his physical abnormalities vanished.

83. Symmetric pulmonary metastases. Although the frontal radiograph resembled that of breast implants, the lateral view clearly placed the lesions in the lungs. At autopsy several weeks later, each lung contained one gigantic metastasis of melanoma. Moreover, the two metastases were remarkably similar in size and shape.

This case could qualify for any list of all-time medical oddities.

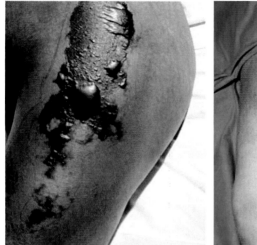
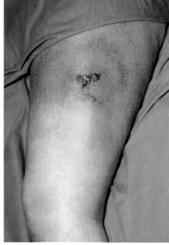

The patient on the left had a deep vein thrombosis, while the patient on the right had rheumatic mitral stenosis with atrial fibrillation.

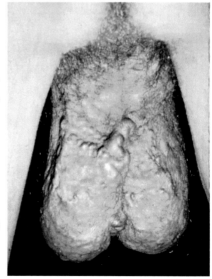

This teenager with Ebstein's anomaly had a pulsatile, murmurless, left-sided scrotal mass.

84 & 85. Coumarin-induced skin necrosis. A rare and unpredictable complication of oral anticoagulation therapy, affecting women more than men. The skin necrosis typically appears on the third to fifth day of therapy, but always within the first two weeks. Frequent areas of involvement are the buttocks, thighs, and breasts. Fingers, hands, neck, and face are typically spared. The pathogenesis remains speculative, but it clearly is not dose-related. Associated congenital or acquired coagulation deficiencies have been identified in a minority of cases. Besides discontinuing anticoagulation therapy, management may include use of Vitamin K, heparin, fibrinolytic agents, or surgical debridement of gangrenous tissue. Depending on the extent and degree of necrosis, the lesions may heal on their own.

86. Pulsating varicocele resulting from tricuspid insufficiency. The prominent scrotal varicosities seen in the image were associated with a large, pulsatile varicocele that initially masqueraded as a pulsating testicle. Other causes of pulsatile scrotal masses include arteriovenous malformation (which has a murmur) and "arteriocele" (a testicular artery that provides a major collateral for an obstructed iliac artery). These conditions are easily differentiated from varicocele by their physical and angiographic features.

The take-home message is this: Pulsating veins, irrespective of their location, are pathognomonic of tricuspid insufficiency.

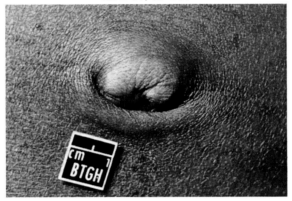

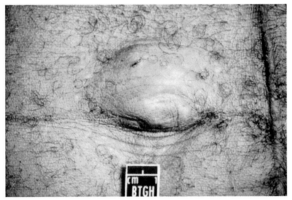

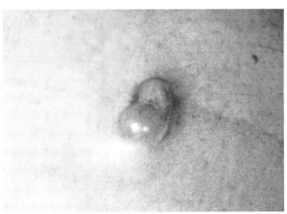

87, 88 & 89. Umbilical metastases. From carcinomas of the pancreas (top), stomach (middle), and ovary(bottom). Umbilical metastases ordinarily occur late in the course of fatal neoplastic disease. Nevertheless, they can be the presenting symptom, earliest sign, or only physical finding of neoplasm arising elsewhere. Although the primary tumor can originate anywhere below the diaphragm, the most commonly reported sites are the stomach and ovary.

Umbilical metastases usually appear as small, irregular, firm, and sometimes painful nodules. Occasionally, however, there may be only thickening and inflammation of the subcutaneous tissue simulating cellulitis or abscess of the umbilicus. Correct diagnosis requires biopsy of the umbilical lesion. The results may spare the patient time, money, and physical and emotional stress.

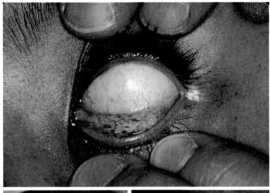

This 25-year-old woman suddenly developed shaking chills, confusion, and a temperature of 103° F. On physical examination, she had numerous petechiae in her palpebral and bulbar conjunctiva (top image) and over the shoulders, arms and upper anterior part of her chest (bottom images).

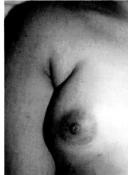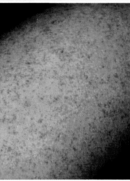

Case 91

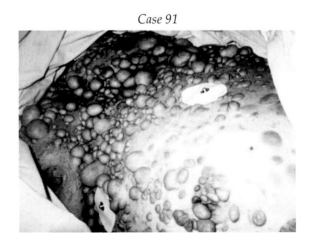

90. Systemic fat embolism. Thirty hours before onset of her fever and chills, this patient fractured her right femur in an auto-pedestrian accident. She ultimately made a full recovery without receiving antibiotics.

In patients with recent fracture of the long bones, the best (and often the first) evidence of systemic fat embolism is the abrupt appearance of petechiae in a characteristic distribution — conjunctivae, base of neck, axillae, and upper anterior part of the arms, shoulders, and chest. If the petechiae develop at all, they usually become visible 24 to 36 hours after the injury. They typically persist for three to four days, then fade rapidly. Their number has no relation to prognosis.

The sudden appearance of fever, chills, and petechiae ordinarily suggests infection, particularly meningococcemia. But if the history indicates recent fracture of a long bone, systemic fat embolism is likely.

91. Neurofibromatosis Type 1. The most common type of neurofibromatosis, affecting about one in 5,000 people. Diagnostic criteria for this autosomal dominant disorder include at least two of the following: 1) six or more café-au-lait spots larger than 5 mm in diameter in children and larger than 15 mm in teenagers and adults; 2) at least two neurofibromas of any type or one plexiform neurofibroma; 3) freckling in the inguinal or axillary regions; 4) optic nerve glioma; 5) two or more iris hamartomas (Lisch nodules); 6) a distinct osseous lesion; and 7) a first-degree relative (parent, sibling, or child) with type 1 neurofibromatosis.

The 45-year-old patient shown had café-au-lait spots noted at birth and neurofibromas noted during puberty. Her mother had similar findings.

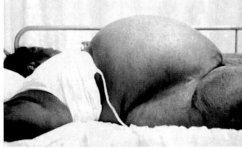

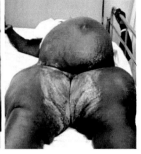

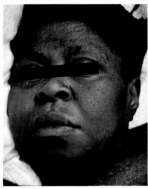

This 56-year-old alcoholic presented with lethargy and increasing abdominal girth of six months' duration. Her admitting diagnosis was hepatic cirrhosis.

Case 93

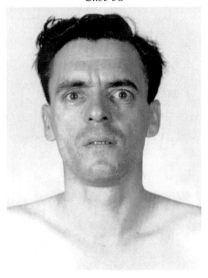

92. Myxedema ascites. This patient's facial features alone were enough to suggest hypothyroidism. In addition, she had a low-pitched voice, dry skin, and pseudomyotonic deep tendon reflexes. After two months of thyroid replacement therapy, she was asymptomatic and looking like her old self again (images below). Liver biopsy at that point showed normal findings.

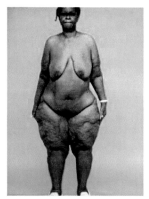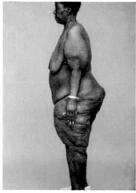

This case emphasizes that alcoholism plus ascites doesn't necessarily equal liver disease.

93. Unilateral thyrotoxic exophthalmos. This 42-year-old man presented with heat intolerance, nervousness, and a 20-lb weight loss of six months' duration. As shown in the image, he had obvious left-sided proptosis and a striking, hawk-like stare bilaterally. He also had visible and palpable enlargement of his thyroid gland, especially the isthmus and right lobe. Laboratory studies confirmed the clinical diagnosis of hyperthyroidism. With radioiodine therapy, the patient became asymptomatic, his thyromegaly resolved, and his exophthalmos all but disappeared.

Two points here deserve emphasis; 1) a prominent stare as seen in this patient should always bring to mind hyperthyroidism; and 2) hyperthyroidism deserves consideration in every patient with unilateral exophthalmos.

Case 94

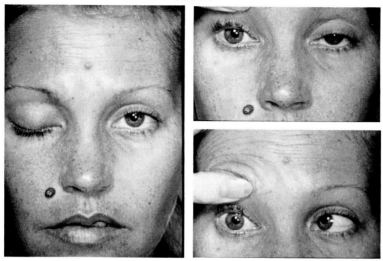

This 25-year-old Caucasian woman complained of progressive headaches, visual difficulties, and darkening of her skin during the preceding six months. Three years earlier, she had undergone bilateral adrenalectomy for treatment of Cushing's disease.

Case 95

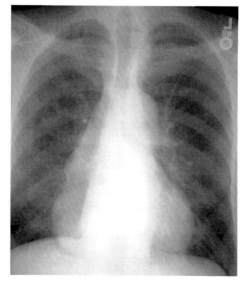

Chest radiograph of a 61-year-old man with a history of long-standing dysphagia and frequent vomiting.

99

94. Nelson's syndrome. Development of an ACTH-producing, rapidly growing, and often invasive pituitary tumor after bilateral adrenalectomy for Cushing's disease. The clinical manifestations are headache, visual field defects, external ophthalmoplegias, and ACTH-induced hyperpigmentation similar to that of Addison's disease.

The patient shown had generalized hyperpigmentation of her skin and mucosal surfaces, a large pituitary mass, bitemporal hemianopia, and palsies of the right 3rd and 6th cranial nerves. After transphenoidal resection of most of her pituitary tumor, coupled with postoperative radiation therapy, her headaches resolved and her vision improved, but her ophthalmoplegias and hyperpigmentation did not change.

95. Achalasia. At first glance, the image suggests cardiomegaly consequent to pericardial effusion or dilated myocardium. On closer inspection, however, the right "heart" border is somewhat irregular and ill-defined. A barium swallow (image below) showed that the abnormal "cardiac" configuration represented a dilated esophagus.

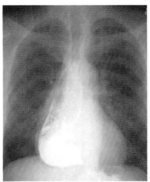

The medical literature appropriately indicates that the dilated esophagus in patients with achalasia can sometimes be mistaken on chest radiographs for mediastinal or pulmonary disease. This case demonstrates that a dilated esophagus can also mimic cardiomegaly.

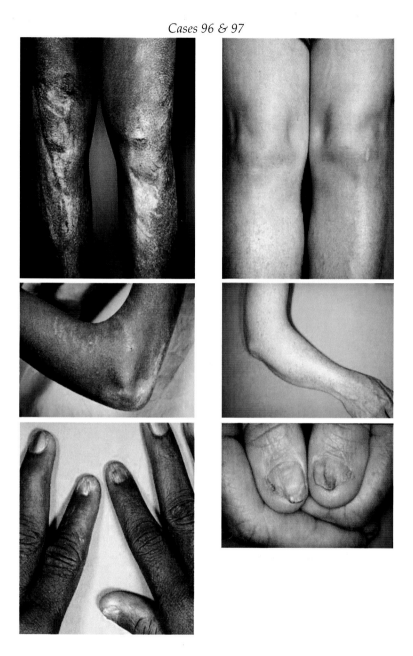

Both of these patients had impaired renal function.

96 & 97. Hereditary osteo-onycho-dysplasia (HOOD).

Also known as the nail-patella syndrome and Fong's disease, this is a genetic disorder of ectodermal and mesodermal tissues characterized by dysplastic nails, deformed elbows, small or absent patellas, and bilateral iliac horns. It is transmitted by an autosomal dominant gene with complete penetrance and variable expressivity, affecting males and females equally. Although the patient on the left is Black, this disorder appears almost exclusively in Caucasians. Renal disease is common and probably constitutes part of the syndrome. Histologically, the kidney shows a variety of cortical and medullary changes.

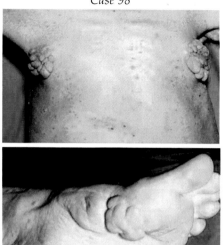

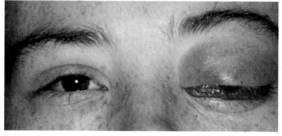

This 25-year-old woman presented with a five-month history of redness, swelling, and blurred vision in her left eye. On examination, the left eyelids were swollen and discolored, the conjunctiva edematous and injected, and the globe moderately proptotic. Studies for neoplasm and infection were negative, and results of thyroid function tests were normal. The radioiodine uptake, however, was not suppressed by administration of triiodothyronine.

98. Neurofibromatosis Type 2. An autosomal dominant disorder affecting about one in 50,000 individuals. Diagnostic criteria for this type include bilateral cranial nerve VIII tumors or a first-degree relative with type 2, and either a unilateral cranial nerve VIII tumor or two of the following: dermal or subcutaneous neurofibromas, plexiform neurofibroma, Schwannoma, glioma, meningioma, or juvenile subcapsular lenticular opacity.

The 43-year-old woman shown had scattered dermal and subcutaneous neurofibromas together with plexiform neurofibromas of both breasts and left foot. Her mother had bilateral cranial nerve VIII tumors.

99. Euthyroid ophthalmic Graves' disease. A form of infiltrative ophthalmopathy characterized by swollen extraocular muscles, increased amounts of retroorbital fat, and absence of toxic goiter. Early symptoms include a sense of irritation in the eyes, excessive tearing, and blurred vision. Exophthalmos, ordinarily bilateral, is the most common finding, along with reddened lids and weakness of the extraocular muscles. The course is variable and unpredictable. Symptomatic care often suffices in mild cases, while glucocorticoids, external radiation, or both are useful in others. For extreme cases, orbital decompression may become necessary.

The patient shown responded promptly but incompletely to large doses of glucocorticoids (image below).

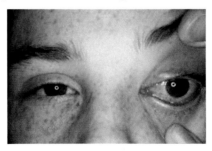

Case 100

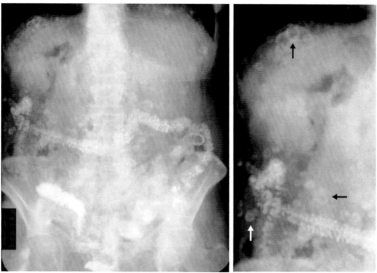

Abdominal radiographs of an elderly woman who, in 1954, underwent a barium enema examination because of recurrent abdominal pain. Scattered throughout the abdomen (left image), particularly in the right subdiaphragmatic area (right image), were numerous, rounded, calcific densities with radiolucent centers (arrows).

Case 101

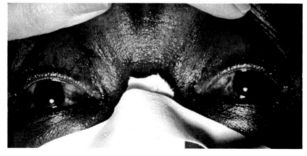

This severely ill 22-year-old man had the abrupt onset of headache, distressing myalgia, shaking chills, and rapid collapse. On examination, he was delirious with a temperature of 104° F.

100. Lipogranuloma of the peritoneum. Also known as oil granuloma, oleoma, oleogranuloma, paraffinoma, vaselinoma of the peritoneum, and "soap bubble syndrome." This patient said that during a cholecystectomy in 1934, the surgeon had poured mineral oil into her peritoneal cavity to prevent adhesions, a practice that began at the turn of the 20th century. The other lipid agents used for this purpose included olive oil, Vaseline, animal fat, and paraffin. With time, however, it became obvious that these substances acted as irritants rather than lubricants. So by the early 1940s or thereabouts, surgeons abandoned this procedure forever.

101. Leptospirosis. Blood from this man grew *Leptospira icterohemorrhagiae*, prompting therapy with high-dose intravenous penicillin. After a course characterized by renal and hepatic failure, the patient ultimately made a full recovery. He presumably became infected through contact with the urine of rats that infested his home.

The diagnostic clue in this case is the combination of icteric sclerae and hemorrhagic conjunctivae; hence the term, "icterohemorrhagiae".

Leptospirosis presents in various ways, from inapparent to fulminating and fatal disease. About 90% of symptomatic patients manifest a mild influenza-like illness that typically resolves uneventfully within two to three weeks. Only a small proportion develop hemorrhagic complications or hepatorenal failure, and of those, only 10% to 20% die.

Case 102

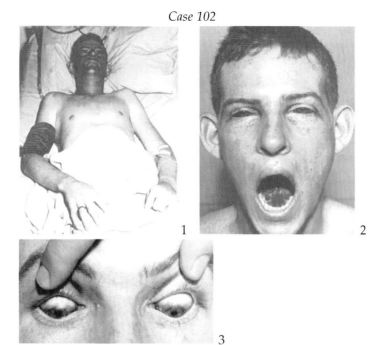

1

2

3

Case 103

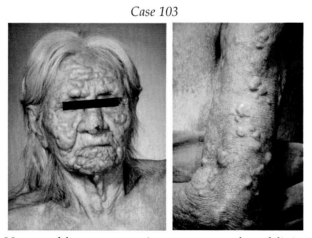

This 90-year-old asymptomatic woman was found living under a bridge. She was unable to supply a reliable medical history.

102. Traumatic asphyxia. This 19-year-old airman sustained a calculated 1400 lbs of pressure to his chest when a stationary jet trainer lost its parked attitude and pinned him to the ground. He was freed within 15 seconds. Observers at the scene noted that his eyes became prominent and that his neck and face turned bright red and then dark blue. Image 1, day 1, shows the bluish-black discoloration of his face and neck. Image 2, day 6, shows massive subconjunctival and sublingual hemorrhages, along with marked clearing of the facial discoloration. Image 3, day 9, shows the typically unaffected portions of the conjunctivae. The skin of the face is now normal. For more information on this condition, see Case 25 on page 35.

103. Leprosy. Hansen's disease, lepromatous type. The patient's facial nodules and plaques, coupled with nodules on her arms and neck, immediately suggested leprosy. A biopsy specimen from a nodule on her arm showed numerous acid-fast organisms in clusters (image below). The rest of her physical examination and results of routine laboratory tests were unremarkable. Subsequently, the patient was transferred to the U.S. Public Health Service Hospital, Carville, Louisiana, for long-term management.

Patients with lepromatous leprosy have no cell-mediated 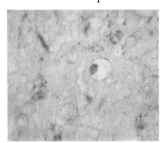 immunity to the causative agent, *Mycobacterium leprae.* Consequently, they have diffuse disease, with many lesions containing large numbers of bacteria. By contrast, patients with tuberculoid leprosy have a high degree of cell-mediated immunity to *M leprae.* As a result, they have localized disease with one or two skin lesions and relatively few bacteria.

One final point. The incubation period for leprosy is uniquely long among bacterial diseases, with a minimum of two to three years, an average of five to seven years, and a maximum of 40 to 50 years.

Case 104

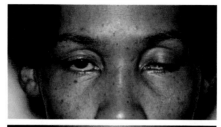

1:00 PM

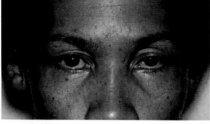

1:02 PM

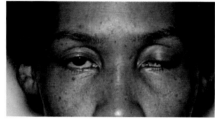

1:09 PM

Case 105

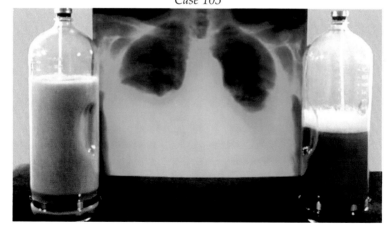

104. Myasthenia gravis. This 25-year-old man presented with bilateral ptosis (greater on the left) and diplopia. He also complained of generalized weakness that worsened as effort increased or as the day progressed.

The images depict the patient showing a positive response to edrophonium chloride (Tensilon). His assay for acetylcholine-receptor antibodies—a test specific for myasthenia gravis—was also positive. He underwent thymectomy (image below) and subsequently functioned well with maintenance corticosteroid therapy.

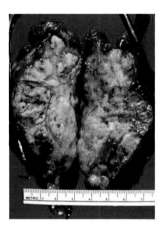

105. Contarini's condition. The term used to indicate bilateral pleural effusions, each with markedly different characteristics and distinctly different mechanisms. It honors Francesco Contarini (1556-1624), the 95th Doge of the Venetian Republic, whose autopsy showed right-sided hydrothorax consequent to heart failure and left-sided empyema presumably resulting from a lung abscess.

The radiograph and pleural fluids shown were from a man with malignant lymphoma that had infiltrated the pleura on the left, causing a bloody effusion, while simultaneously obstructing the thoracic duct on the right, causing a chylous effusion.

Case 106

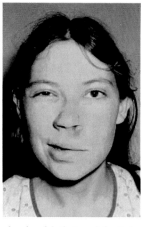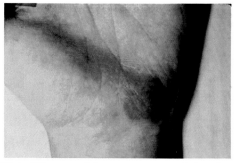

This 22-year-old woman complained of difficulty smiling, weakness of her hands, and bumps on her skin of two months' duration. On examination, she had bilateral facial weakness (more prominent on the left), a left abducens weakness, and bilateral ulnar palsies. She also had red, indurated papular lesions on her left hypothenar eminence and abutting her nose. The skin lesions were anesthetic and showed granulomatous inflammation on biopsy.

Case 107

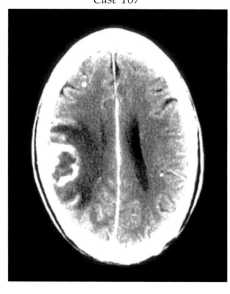

Contrast-enhanced cranial CT scan of a 42-year-old HIV-positive man with numbness and weakness in his left hand. He denied headaches, fever, mental change, visual difficulty, or speech disturbance. His spinal fluid had 21 leukocytes per mm^3, 118 mg/dL of protein, and a VDRL reactive 1:4. Various stains and cultures of the fluid were negative.

111

106. Lymphomatoid granulomatosis. The clinical findings in this patient initially suggested sarcoidosis, then leprosy. But after extensive study at two university medical centers and the Public Health Service Hospital at Carville, Louisiana, the final diagnosis was lymphomatoid granulomatosis—a disease with features resembling those of lymphoma and Wegener's granulomatosis. Histologically, the characteristic finding is a granulomatous process with a polymorphous lymphoreticular infiltration, angiocentric and angiodestructive in nature, with atypical and occasionally bizarre lymphohistiocytic cells.

Although virtually any organ can be affected by this disease, pulmonary, neurologic, and cutaneous manifestations predominate. No consistently effective therapy has been established, and the prognosis is poor.

In the patient shown, the skin lesions resolved with corticosteroid therapy, but the neurologic difficulties worsened. After a year of illness, she had become paraplegic. Curiously, no evidence of pulmonary disease ever emerged during that time.

107. Cerebral gumma. The ring-enhancing lesion with surrounding edema in the right parietal lobe was consistent with neoplasm, opportunistic infection, and pyogenic abscess. But the spinal fluid findings indicated active neurosyphilis with probable gumma formation. Accordingly, the patient received high-dose penicillin intravenously for 21 days. On day 16 of therapy, a repeat CT scan showed that the brain lesion had all but disappeared. And by day 21, the patient was asymptomatic with a normal physical examination.

Despite their relative rarity, cerebral gummata deserve consideration in patients who have one or more brain masses and laboratory evidence of syphilis. On CT scan, the cerebral gumma typically appears as a peripherally located, contrast-enhancing lesion, with or without surrounding edema. Therefore, it can be easily mistaken for neoplasm, abscess, opportunistic infection, or infarct.

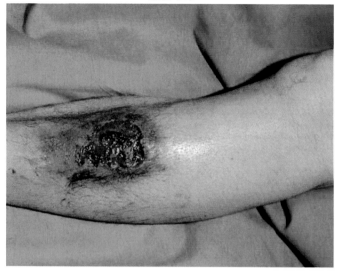

The lower leg of a 30-year-old man with ulcerative colitis.

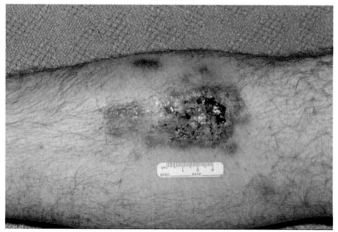
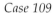

The lower leg of a 37-year-old man who injured it while gardening. Two weeks later, a small ulcer appeared at the injury site and slowly expanded during the next month. The lesion did not improve with antibiotic therapy.

108. Pyoderma gangrenosum. A disorder of uncertain cause that may appear on any mucocutaneous surface but has a predilection for the lower extremities. Of the four main clinical variants—ulcerative, pustular, bullous, and vegetative—the ulcerative form is the most prevalent. Along with the pustular variant, the ulcerative form is associated most frequently with active inflammatory bowel disease. The bullous and vegetative types generally occur with myelodysplastic and lymphoproliferative disorders.

The diagnosis is usually made clinically. Serologic, hematologic, and histopathologic findings are nonspecific. Differential diagnosis includes a wide variety of infections as well as insect or spider bites, drug reactions, vasculitis, and the antiphospholipid-antibody syndrome. Corticosteroids are the mainstay of treatment and often control and sometimes cure the lesion. Acceptable therapeutic alternatives are dapsone, bactrim, clofazimine, and minocycline. Because trauma can intensify the inflammatory process, debridement is contra-indicated

109. Lymphocutaneous sporotrichosis. A dermatologist saw this patient initially and diagnosed pyoderma gangrenosum. But he only examined the lower leg. Had he examined the entire leg, he might have noticed the telltale nodular lymphangitis in the right thigh (image below) — a further clue to sporo-

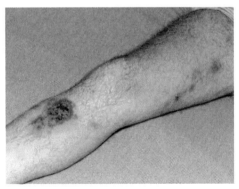

trichosis in this gardener. Culture of the lesion subsequently grew *Sporothrix schencki*.

Other organisms that cause nodular lymphangitis after cutaneous inoculation include *Nocardia brasiliensis*, *Mycobacterium marinum*, *Leishmania brasiliensis*, and *Francisella tularensis*.

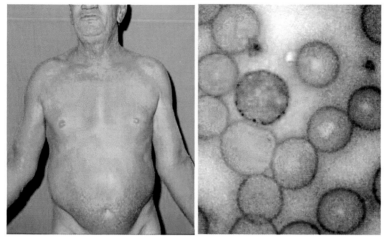

This 61-year-old man presented in 1972 with unrelenting pruritus of six months' duration. On the right is his peripheral blood film stained with Periodic Acid-Schiff (PAS).

Case 111

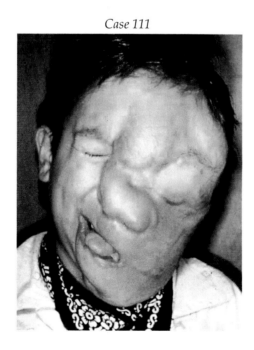

110. Sézary syndrome (SS). A rare form of cutaneous lymphoma characterized by intractable pruritus, generalized erythroderma, diffuse lymphadenopathy, and neoplastic T cells (Sézary cells) in the skin, lymph nodes, and peripheral blood. The Sézary cells in the blood are mononuclear, usually numerous, and have round or oval nuclei with densely clumped chromatin. They often stain intensely with PAS (image below), but more sophisticated techniques are now available to identify them.

SS predominantly affects men over the age of 60. When the erythroderma is generalized, the term *l'homme rouge* (the red man) has been applied. Treatment currently includes photophoresis, with or without interferon, chemotherapy, and total skin electron beam therapy. Prognosis is poor with a median survival of two to four years.

The patient shown received prednisone and systemic chemotherapy. His skin manifestations initially improved, but he subsequently manifested widespread lymphadenopathy with hepatosplenomegaly and died four years after onset of symptoms.

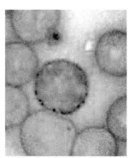

111. Neurofibromatosis Type 2. In addition to his facial disfigurement, this 10-year-old boy had a few large neurofibromas and café-au-lait spots on his neck and back. Most impressive, however, was this youngster's magnetic personality. Despite a physical appearance that ordinarily would prompt a reclusive lifestyle, he was a happy-go-lucky, inspiring child whom everyone admired.

Case 112

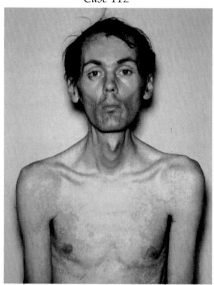

This 40-year-old man presented with bilateral cataracts and complete heart block.

Case 113

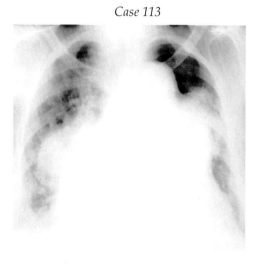

Chest radiograph of a 63-year-old, critically ill woman with an elevated jugular venous pressure, hyperdynamic precordium, and grade IV/VI systolic and diastolic murmurs heard best to the left of the sternum at the third and fourth interspaces. Her electrocardiogram showed atrial fibrillation and a pattern of right ventricular hypertrophy.

112. Myotonic dystrophy. An autosomal dominant form of muscular dystrophy characterized by abnormally prolonged muscle contraction after active motion or mechanical stimulation. Typical associated features are frontal alopecia; lens opacities; atrophy of the temporalis, zygomaticus, and sternocleidomastoid muscles; and gonadal atrophy in men. Widespread smooth muscle involvement may also cause cardiac conduction disturbances and arrhythmias, esophageal and colonic dysfunction, and respiratory disability.

The patient shown had early frontal balding, wasting of his temporal and facial muscles, and virtually no visible neck or shoulder muscles. His inability to immediately relax his grip after the introductory handshake sealed the diagnosis.

113. Aneurysmal dilatation of the main pulmonary arteries. On hospital day two, right heart catheterization disclosed a pulmonary arterial pressure of 98/35 mm Hg (mean, 60

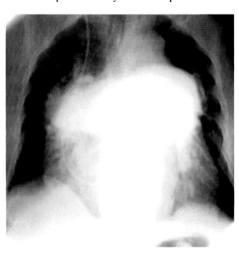

mm Hg), and angiography demonstrated massive dilatation of the major pulmonary arteries (image at left). The next day, the patient died. Autopsy disclosed aneurysmal dilatation of the main pulmonary arteries and a healed dissecting aneurysm extending from the arch of the aorta to the iliac bifurcation. Cystic medial necrosis (CMN) was evident throughout the pulmonary arterial tree as well as the aorta and its major branches.

CMN characteristically affects the aorta. That it may also involve the pulmonary vasculature is not widely appreciated.

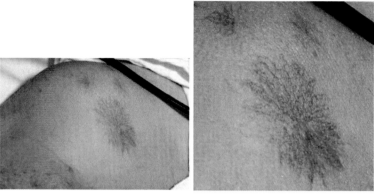

This 47-year-old patient had longstanding jaundice and ascites consequent to biopsy-proven hepatic cirrhosis.

Case 115

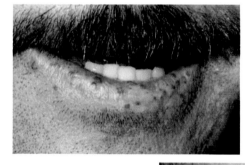

Case 116

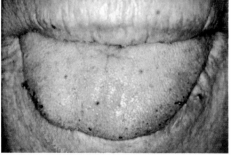

114. Gigantic cutaneous arterial spiders. Although arterial spiders vary in size and shape, most are less than 1 to 2 cm in greatest diameter. In the patient shown, however, several spiders on his abdomen were unusually large, the largest being 7x14 cm.

115 & 116 Hereditary hemorrhagic telangiectasia. Osler-Weber-Rendu disease. An autosomal dominant systemic fibrovascular dysplasia in which varying numbers of telangiectases, arteriovenous malformations, and aneurysms appear throughout the body. The manifestations are diverse and stem directly from these vascular abnormalities in the nose, skin, lung, brain, and gastrointestinal tract. Hemorrhage and anemia are the two most frequent consequences.

The clinical hallmark of this disease—illustrated by the two patients shown—is the telangiectasis, a focal dilatation of postcapillary venules. These bright red to purple lesions range in size from pinpoint to about 3 mm in diameter, are flat, blanch on pressure, and increase in number with age. They occur most commonly on the face, lips, tongue, ears, conjunctivae, palms, and soles.

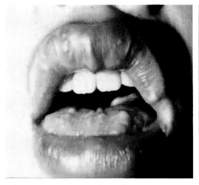 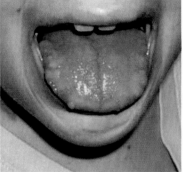

These two unrelated patients—a 14-year-old boy (left) and a 23-year-old woman (right)—have the same disease.

This 40-year-old man com-plained of puffy eyes, dry skin, and muscle stiffness of six months' duration.

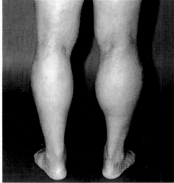 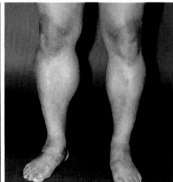

117 & 118. Multiple endocrine neoplasia, Type IIB (MEN-IIB). An inherited, autosomal dominant disease characterized by medullary thyroid carcinoma, pheochromocytoma, and mucosal neuromas, associated at times with prognathism, puffy lips, and bony abnormalities. Both of these patients had surgically treated medullary thyroid carcinoma, neuromas of the tongue and lips, and prognathism. Neither, however, had any evidence, as yet, of adrenal disease.

119. Hypothyroid myopathy. Hoffmann's syndrome. In addition to puffy eyelids and dry skin, this patient had a markedly delayed relaxation phase of his deep tendon reflexes and prominent enlargement of his right calf. On palpation, the calf was firm but not tender. These physical findings prompted thyroid hormone replacement therapy, and within six months, all of the aforementioned abnormalities disappeared.

Hoffman's syndrome refers to varying degrees of weakness, muscle stiffness, and increased muscle mass in adults with severe hypothyroidism. The cause of the increased muscle mass awaits clarification. On histopathologic examination, the involved muscles have densely packed fibers with variable diameters and loss of normal striations. One or both calf muscles are among the more commonly involved sites, but almost any muscle group may be affected. Thyroid hormone therapy is curative.

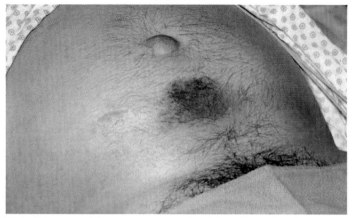

This 36-year-old man presented with a four-day history of severe epigastric pain following an alcoholic binge. His serum amylase level was 821 U/L, and an abdominal CT scan showed marked inflammatory changes in his pancreas, omentum, and surrounding mesentery.

Case 121

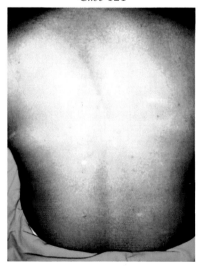

This 14-year-old boy had a lifelong history of mental retardation and epilepsy.

120. Acute pancreatitis with Cullen's sign. In patients with acute pancreatitis, ecchymoses of the abdominal wall may appear near the midline anywhere from the umbilicus to the symphysis pubis (Cullen's sign). These ecchymoses, however, are not specific for pancreatitis, and in the absence of trauma and blood disorders, merely signal retroperitoneal or intra-abdominal hemorrhage.

121. Hypomelanotic ("ash-leaf") macules of tuberous sclerosis. Also known as Bournville disease and epiloia, this multisystem, autosomal dominant disorder has a wide variety of manifestations, chief of which are skin abnormalities, tonic-clonic seizures, and mental retardation.

The hypomelanotic macules (arrows, image at left) are pathognomonic of tuberous sclerosis. They are the earliest and most common cutaneous sign, occurring in almost 90% of the

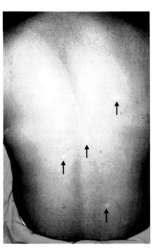

patients. Usually evident at birth or during the first year of life, these lesions may involve any part of the body's surface, vary in number from four to 100, typically exceed 1 cm in diameter, are dull-white in color, and are lance-oval in shape (tapered at one end and round at the other— the same shape as that of leaflets from the mountain-ash tree).

Other pathognomonic skin lesions of tuberous sclerosis generally appear years later and include adenoma sebaceum on the face, shagreen (shark-skin) patches in the lumbar area, and periungual and gingival fibromas.

Case 122

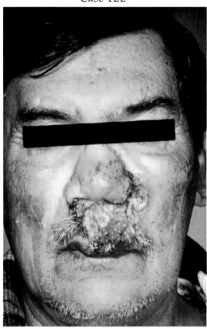

This 61-year-old man presented with a four-month history of progressively destructive disease of his mid-face. He had no associated signs or symptoms, and his oral cavity and facial bones were not involved. His nasal septum, however, was perforated.

Case 123

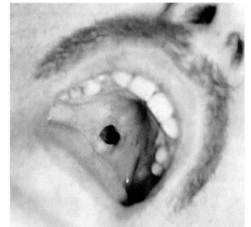

This 42-year-old cocaine addict complained of long-standing nasal stuffiness and recurrent epistaxis. On examination, he had crusting and ulceration of the nasal mucosa, perforation of the nasal septum, and a hole in his soft palate.

122. Lethal midline granuloma. The term used at the time of the patient's presentation (1965) to describe inflammatory destructive lesions of unknown cause. With the sophisticated testing available today, however, most of these patients are now known to have lymphoma or Wegener's granulomatosis. Other documented causes of this "midline granuloma" syndrome include cocaine abuse; trauma; certain bacterial, fungal, and parasitic infections; malignant neoplasms; connective tissue diseases; sarcoidosis; and hypersensitivity angiitis.

The lesion shown healed completely after local radiotherapy (image below), and the patient remained free of disease during a three-year follow-up.

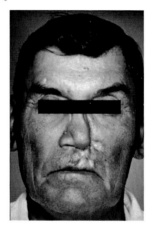

123. Cocaine-induced midline destructive lesion.
Compulsive nasal insufflation of pulverized cocaine can damage the nasal mucosa and lead to ischemic necrosis of the septal cartilage and ultimate perforation of the nasal septum. The same mechanism presumably accounts for the palatal abnormality shown in the image. Differentiating these cocaine-induced lesions from those of limited Wegener's granulomatosis can be difficult, particularly if the patient does not readily admit to substance abuse.

Lateral chest radiograph of a 15-year-old boy who experienced acute pleurisy following a severe bout of vomiting.

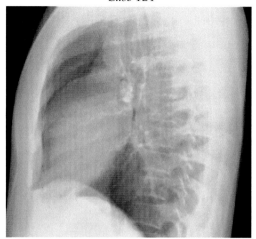

Case 125

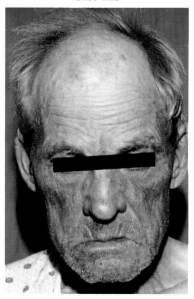

This 64-year-old man presented with a four-month history of episodic wheezing and diarrhea. His wife said that when they dined together, she noticed that his cheeks would become flushed and remain so for about an hour after the meal. The patient was symptom-free during these times.

124. The "ring around the artery" sign. Air surrounding the right pulmonary artery (arrows, image below) has been documented in only a few cases and is diagnostic of pneumomediastinum. It is best seen on the lateral projection and may be the only radiographic evidence of pneumomediastinum.

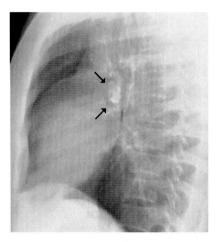

125. Carcinoid syndrome. In addition to his facial flushing, this patient had facial telangiectases, an enlarged liver, and striking murmurs of tricuspid regurgitation and pulmonic stenosis. A liver biopsy specimen showed a neuroendocrine tumor with characteristics indicative of a midgut carcinoid.

This case illustrates several important clinical features of the carcinoid syndrome:
1) right-sided valvular heart lesions are characteristic and offer an immediate clue to the diagnosis;
2) with few exceptions, hepatic metastases have already occurred by the time flushing first appears;
3) the flushes can vary considerably in color, frequency, duration, distribution, and symptomatology;
4) eating provokes the flushing in some patients.

Cases 126, 127 & 128

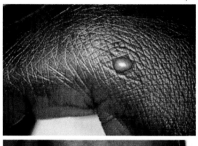
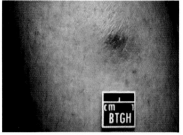

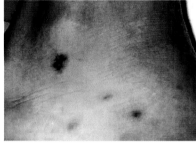

Acral skin lesions of three young adults with fever and painful joints of several days' duration.

Case 129

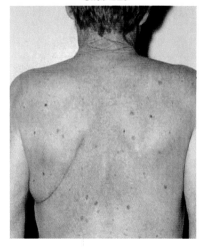

126, 127 & 128. Gonococcal dermatitis. A characteristic eruption accompanying transient gonococcal bacteremia. The lesions are discrete, scanty, 1 mm to 2 cm in diameter, and typically appear on the distal parts of the extremities, often periarticular. They begin as erythematous macules and quickly become vesiculopustular or hemorrhagic. Occasionally, bullae develop. Mature lesions are elevated and slightly umbilicated and have a gray, necrotic center with an irregular violaceous border. Healing occurs in three to four days, with or without therapy.

129. The Sign of Leser-Trélat. A cutaneous marker of internal malignancy described in the 19th century by two surgeons, Edmund Leser (German) and Ulysse Trélat (French). This sign refers to the sudden appearance and rapid increase in size and number of seborrheic keratoses on skin that was previously blemish-free. In most of the reported cases, adenocarcinoma has been the commonest tissue type, while the gastrointestinal tract has been the commonest site of origin. Other tissue types have included leukemias, lymphomas, sarcomas, and squamous cell carcinomas.

The seborrheic keratoses may precede, accompany, or follow detection of the primary tumor and may regress or disappear when the primary tumor is treated. Why these keratoses appear remains speculative.

In the patient shown, squamous cell carcinoma of the lung was the primary tumor. Note the thoracotomy scar beneath the left scapula.

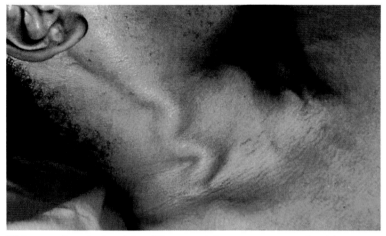

This previously healthy 39-year-old man presented with congestive heart failure of recent onset.

Case 131

The lesion on the neck of this homeless man had been slowly enlarging for 18 months, unaccompanied by fever, weight loss, or other systemic signs. On examination, the lesion was hard and nodular with redness of the overlying skin; however, it was not painful, tender, or warm. There were no other physical abnormalities, and results of conventional laboratory tests were normal. Findings from computed tomography (CT) of the neck were interpreted as those of an abscess. The same study

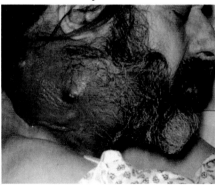

performed on the patient at another hospital one year earlier had prompted the same interpretation. Yet no infection was established at that time, and the patient had left the hospital before any therapy could be administered.

130. Traumatic arteriovenous (AV) fistula. Twenty years before manifesting heart failure, this patient sustained a stab wound to his neck. He recovered on his own and remained well until the current illness began.

Even without that history, the size and tortuosity of the neck vein displayed in the image strongly suggested an AV fistula. A palpable thrill and a continuous murmur were evident over the vein. Moreover, compressing the vein abolished the murmur and decreased the heart rate from 110 beats/min to 80 beats/min (Branham's sign). An arteriogram showed a connection between the right external carotid artery and the right external jugular vein. Surgical closure of the fistula resulted in resolution of the patient's high-output heart failure.

131. Squamous cell carcinoma. Site of origin unknown. Given this patient's indolent course and absence of systemic manifestations, the main diagnostic considerations were malignancy vs. chronic infection, particularly actinomycosis or tuberculosis. Surgical biopsy of the lesion settled the issue.

This case illustrates an important point — as with all tests, CT can be misinterpreted and consequently misleading.

Case 132

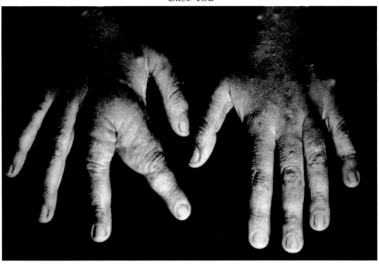

Case 133

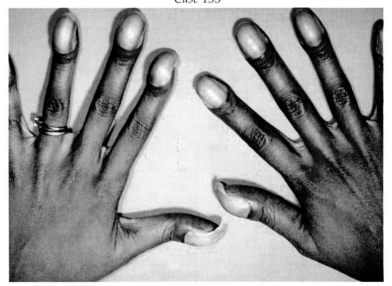

This 18-year-old, healthy-appearing, asymptomatic woman had cyanotic nail beds.

132. Neurofibromatosis Type 1. This patient's mother also had neurofibromatosis. For more information on this disorder, see Case 91 on page 95.

133. Congenital cyanotic heart disease. Digital clubbing with cyanotic nail beds in an otherwise healthy-appearing, asymptomatic young adult is characteristic of a congenital cardiac anomaly with right-to-left shunting. The patient shown had tetralogy of Fallot, the most common congenital cyanotic heart disease in adults.

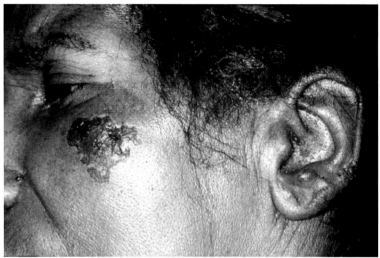

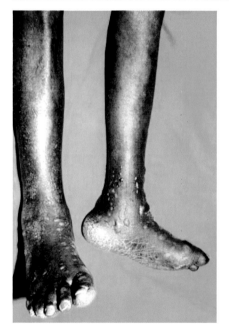

This 50-year-old woman presented with painful necrotic lesions on her left cheek and left ear. She also had livedo reticularis on both lower legs and early gangrene with blistering of both feet. Her carotid and pedal pulses were strong.

Laboratory findings at admission included a normocytic anemia with unremarkable leukocyte and platelet counts, rouleaux formation on the peripheral blood film, 3+ proteinuria, and an elevated serum creatinine level.

134. Multiple myeloma with Type I cryoglobulinemia.
Because this patient had strong carotid and pedal pulses, the necrosis of her cheek and ear together with early gangrene of her feet indicated microvascular occlusions. And since her initial laboratory findings suggested multiple myeloma, the possibility of associated cryoglobulinemia immediately came to mind. Subsequent studies confirmed both diagnoses.

Cryoglobulins are proteins—most commonly immunoglobulins—that precipitate, crystallize, or gel when cooled but redissolve when warmed. They are classified as follows: Type I, a monoclonal protein occurring most often in multiple myeloma but also in B-cell neoplasms; Type II, a mixture of monoclonal and polyclonal proteins; and Type III, consisting solely of polyclonal proteins.

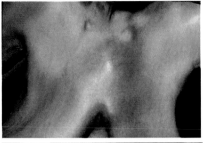

135

This 42-year-old woman had generalized lymphadenopathy, hepatosplenomegaly, and several hard, nonpainful, sternal masses.

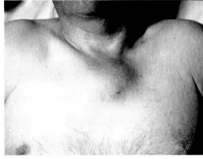

136

This 60-year-old man had hematuria and a pulsatile sternal mass.

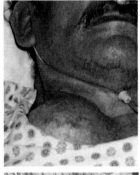

137

This 63-year-old man had a large, rounded, nontender, firm mass in the area of the right sternoclavicular joint. He was afebrile but had anemia, proteinuria, and renal insufficiency.

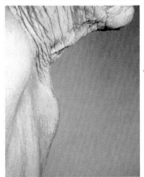

138

This 76-year-old woman presented with jaundice and a mass in the upper part of her sternum.

135. Hodgkin's disease. Involving the sternum.

136. Renal cell carcinoma. Metastatic to the sternum.

137. Multiple myeloma. With plasmacytoma involving the right sternoclavicular joint.

138. Pancreatic carcinoma. Metastatic to the sternum.

Most sternal masses represent metastases. The primary tumor is usually lymphoma, multiple myeloma, or carcinoma of the breast, kidney, or thyroid. Pulsation of the mass strongly suggests multiple myeloma or metastases from renal or thyroid carcinoma.

Primary sternal tumors almost always are malignant and typically are chondrosarcomas.

In some cases, sternal swelling signals infection (e.g., tuberculosis, coccidioidomycosis, aspergillosis, brucellosis, and staphylococcal or pseudomonal disease).

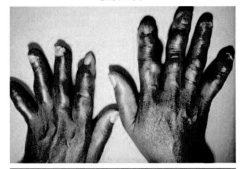

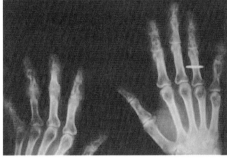

This 36-year-old man presented with a two-year history of swelling and limited motion of both hands. On examination, the fingers were swollen, nontender, and boggy to palpation, with normal overlying skin. The interphalangeal joints moved little, if at all, but the wrists and metacarpophalangeal joints were normal. No other bone or joint disease was evident.

Radiographically, cystic destructive lesions affected most of the phalanges of both hands; the interphalangeal joint spaces were narrowed as well.

Case 140

This 47-year-old woman presented with a swollen and minimally tender right thumb. She felt fine otherwise and had no additional complaints.

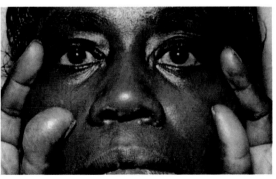

139. Advanced phalangeal sarcoidosis. In addition to his abnormal hands, this patient had bilateral hilar enlargement on chest radiograph and biopsy-proven sarcoidal facial papules.

The incidence of osseous sarcoidosis ranges from 2% to 30% in most series. Although any bone can be affected, the hands and feet are the most frequent sites. Of the various radiographic features, lytic lesions predominate. Other findings include thickening of cortical bone with a fine, lacy, reticular alteration of the trabecular pattern, sclerosis of the distal phalanges, and gross destruction of the bone and joint.

Most bony involvement in sarcoidosis is asymptomatic and requires no treatment. If, however, pain, disability, or deformity becomes an issue, corticosteroid therapy can ease the discomfort and, in some cases, promote healing.

The differential diagnosis includes gout and granulomatous infections such as tuberculosis and fungal disease.

140. Cutaneous sarcoidosis with sarcoidal dactylitis. The papules on and around this patient's nares, and those on her upper eyelids near the inner canthus, strongly suggested sarcoidosis. A radiograph of her affected right thumb demonstrated a lytic lesion in the tip of the distal phalanx. Biopsies of that lesion and a nasal papule showed noncaseating granulomas containing multinucleated giant cells typical of sarcoidosis.

This case illustrates an important clinical point: When bone lesions occur in patients with sarcoidosis, chronic sarcoidal skin changes are almost always present as well.

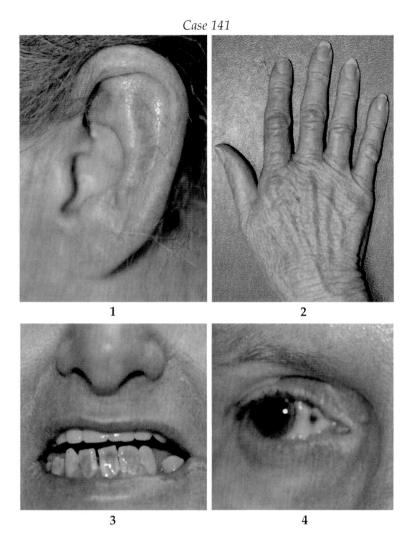

1

2

3

4

This 52-year-old woman had a lifelong history of passing dark urine. At presentation, she was wheelchair-bound because of longstanding and progressively severe knee and back pain.

141. Alcaptonuria with ochronosis. Alcaptonuria is a rare inherited metabolic disease in which absence of the enzyme homogentisic acid oxidase results in excessive amounts of homogentisic acid in the urine. If such urine is alkaline on voiding, is made alkaline, or is simply left standing, its color becomes brown to black throughout.

Ochronosis is the condition in which a brown-black pigment is deposited in connective tissues of the body, especially cartilage, and to a lesser extent, skin and sclera. In most cases, the pigment is a derivative of homogentisic acid, but in a few instances the pigment results from long-term contact with phenol compounds, from industrial contact with quinones, or from use of quinacrine.

The patient shown had the classic bluish discoloration of the cartilage in her ears (image 1), subtle bluish discoloration of the skin overlying the knuckles and tendons of her hands (image 2), and a bluish hue of the tip of her nose and of her teeth (image 3). She also had a typical ochronotic brown-black spot on her right sclera (image 4).

Radiographs of her spine (image 5) showed the telltale sign of ochronotic spondylosis—diffuse calcification of the intervertebral discs. And radiographs of her knees (image 6) showed characteristic degenerative changes in the cartilage, leading to narrowed joint space with advanced eburnation of the opposing bone surfaces.

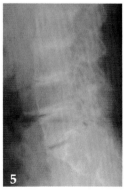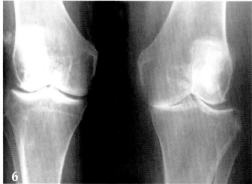

Case 142

This 40-year-old homosexual man presented with weakness, weight loss, and painless, nonpruritic facial lesions of six weeks'

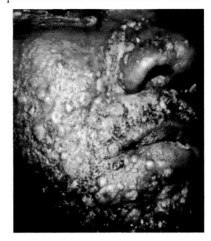

duration. Similar skin changes were present over his legs and lower trunk. On physical examination, the lesions were papulopustular, round or oval, and sharply demarcated. They varied in size from a few millimeters to several centimeters. Many were umbilicated, some ulcerated, and a few crusted. The mucous membranes were normal.

Case 143

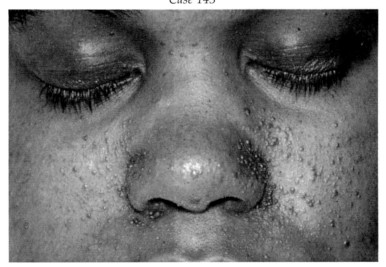

This 17-year-old mentally retarded girl had tonic-clonic seizures since childhood.

142. Malignant syphilis. Also known as syphilis maligna praecox and lues maligna, this is a rare but completely reversible variant of secondary syphilis. Although its incidence had been decreasing since the beginning of the 20th century, the number of reported cases has increased of late, most of them in patients with HIV infection. The skin lesions are pleomorphic, appear in various stages of development, and become widespread, affecting the face and scalp most often. They begin as papulopustules, rapidly undergo necrosis, and tend to form deep crusts. Mucous membranes are involved in about a third of the cases. Histologic examination shows dense infiltrates of plasma cells and histiocytes along with obliterative vasculitis of medium-sized vessels. Spirochetes may be visible in the tissue sections, under dark field microscopy, or both. In addition, a reactive serologic test for syphilis, sometimes with very high titers, is the rule.

The differential diagnosis includes fungal infection, leishmaniasis, verrucous sarcoidosis, bartonellosis, leprosy, yaws, mycosis fungoides, and pyoderma gangrenosum.

The patient shown had positive serologic tests for syphilis, and after three weeks of penicillin therapy, his skin lesions resolved completely.

143. Tuberous sclerosis. A hereditary condition transmitted in an autosomal dominant fashion with variable expressivity. Shown in the image are the pathognomonic facial angiofibromas (adenoma sebaceum) that occur in about 50% of these patients.

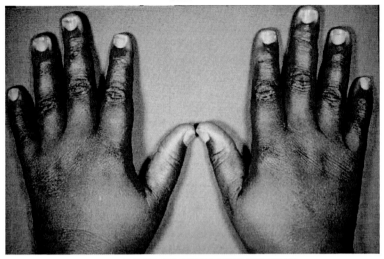

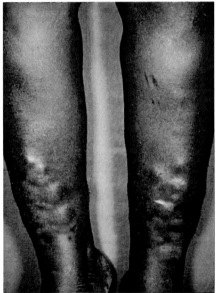

This 33-year-old woman presented with painless swelling of her fingers and lower legs of about four months' duration.

144. Pretibial myxedema and thyroid acropachy accompanying hyperthyroidism.

On physical examination, this patient was thyrotoxic with bilateral exophthalmos and a diffusely enlarged thyroid gland (image below).

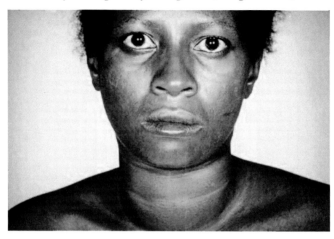

Localized myxedema—disposition of mucopolysaccharides in the skin—typically occurs in the pretibial area. Rarely, however, such deposits can affect the hands, arms, face, ears, shoulders, back, or abdomen. The myxedema ordinarily develops after the diagnosis of thyrotoxicosis has been established but occasionally occurs before or with other clinical signs of hyperthyroidism. Associated ophthalmopathy is almost invariable. Treatment with plasmapheresis, cytotoxic agents, and topically applied corticosteroids is moderately effective, but complete remission occurs in only about 10% of the cases.

Acropachy is a rare manifestation of thyroid disease and nearly always is associated with past or present hyperthyroidism, exophthalmos, and pretibial myxedema. It is characterized by soft-tissue swelling of phalanges, clubbing of terminal phalanges, and periosteal new bone formation in the hands and feet. This condition usually causes no pain or disability and requires no specific treatment.

Case 145

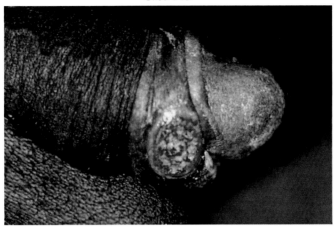

Case 146

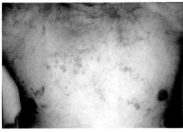

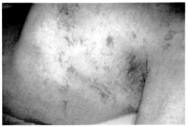

This 60-year-old man presented with a two-week history of hemoptysis. Four months earlier, he had noticed the onset of numerous small, painless, bluish discolorations all over the anterolateral portions of his chest. He assumed they were bruises.

145. Syphilitic chancre. The primary stage of infection with the spirochete *Treponema pallidum*. Ten to 90 days after exposure, the chancre appears at the site of innoculation—usually the anogenital area but sometimes the lip, tongue, or tonsil. It begins as a maculopapule, undergoes ischemic necrosis, and ends up with raised, smooth, sharply defined borders. The lesion is painless and ranges from 0.3 cm to 2 cm in diameter. It heals spontaneously in 4 -14 weeks or within a week or so when treated.

Finding spirochetes under dark field microscopy or obtaining positive serologic tests for syphilis confirms the diagnosis. The differential diagnosis includes chancroid, granuloma inguinale, lymphogranuloma venereum, and penile carcinoma.

In the patient shown, dark field microscopy was positive and response to therapy was rapid and complete.

146. Venous stars heralding superior vena caval syndrome. On physical examination, this man had the full-blown picture of superior vena caval obstruction, proven at autopsy one month later to result from bronchogenic carcinoma. Particularly striking were the many small, dilated, superficial, cutaneous veins—called "venous stars"—that constituted the first objective evidence of mediastinal disease.

Ordinarily, venous stars are not clinically significant. They occur commonly over the thighs, lower legs, dorsum of the feet, and ankles. Moreover, they are frequent along the lower borders of the ribs, in the lower lumbar and upper sacral regions, and over the back, particularly at the junction of the neck and thorax. But when they suddenly appear in the anterolateral thoracic area, they strongly suggest a recent occlusion of one or more of the great thoracic veins.

This is the heart of a 38-year-old, previously healthy, asymptomatic woman who suddenly collapsed and died while watching TV.

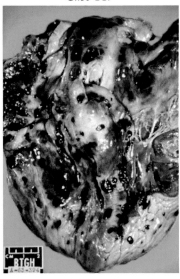

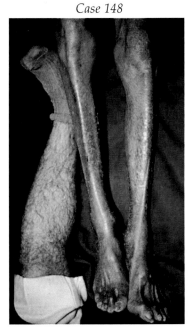

This 62-year-old Caucasian diabetic said that his skin was slowly getting darker. On examination, he had an enlarged, firm liver and diffusely hyperpigmented skin with a deep bronze tint, especially prominent over the legs. (The intern's leg serves as control.)

147. Metastatic melanoma. Autopsy of this patient disclosed extensive metastases not only to her heart, but also to her liver and intestines (image below). The site of the primary melanoma was never established. Death undoubtedly resulted from an arrhythmia.

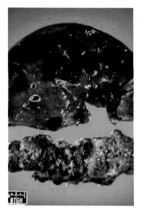

Cardiac metastases ordinarily are clinically silent. But when signs or symptoms do occur, pericardial effusion (with or without tamponade) and dysrhythmias are the most common presentations. Cardiac failure, however, as well as superior vena caval syndrome and other manifestations related to intracavitary metastases, may develop as well.

From a percentage standpoint, melanoma is the most frequent neoplasm metastasizing to the heart (about 65%). Furthermore, the absolute amount of tumor deposited in the heart in cases of melanoma is far greater than that of any other cancer. In one reported case, for example, the melanoma-infiltrated heart weighed 2450 gm! Findings of this sort have given rise to the term "charcoal heart."

148. Hemochromatosis. This case is a classic example of "bronzed diabetes." The patient had elevated serum levels of iron and ferritin, along with increased transferrin saturation. His liver biopsy showed cirrhosis with excessive iron.

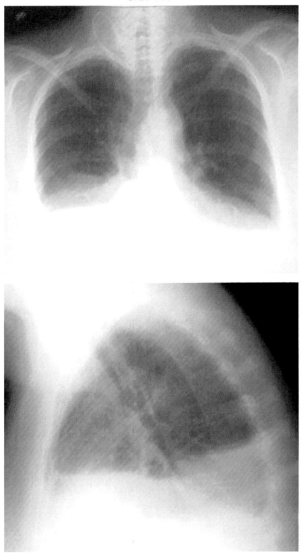

This previously healthy 49-year-old woman underwent a cholecystectomy and repair of a perforated duodenum. On postoperative day seven, her complaints of cough and shortness of breath prompted the radiographs shown above. Despite diuretic therapy, her condition deteriorated, and she died three days later, severely hypoxic and undiagnosed.

149. Vascular erosion by a central venous catheter.
On close inspection of the lateral radiograph (image below), a central venous catheter (arrows) is visible behind the sternum, with the tip far from its intended position near the right atrium. With the catheter tip clearly extravascular, the infusate presumably dripped directly into the chest cavity rather than into the right atrium. Autopsy disclosed large amounts of serous fluid in each pleural space, but the heart, lungs, pulmonary arteries, and other body organs were unremarkable.

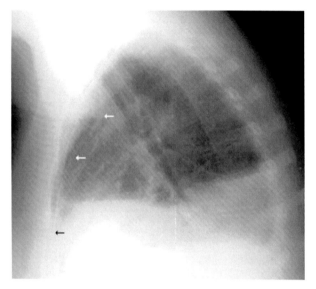

This case teaches several important lessons:

1) when a patient with an indwelling central venous catheter develops new or progressive cardiorespiratory distress, vascular erosion or perforation deserves immediate consideration;
2) a lateral radiograph of the chest can be the best way to verify a malpositioned central venous catheter;
3) failure to recognize this complication can prove fatal.

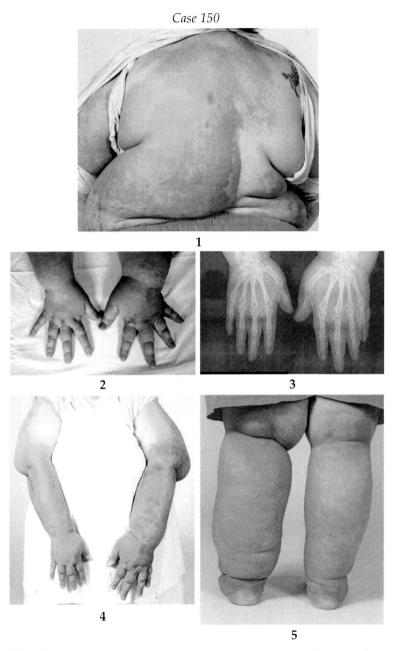

1

2

3

4

5

This 42-year-old woman was asymptomatic except for lymph-edema in both lower legs.

150. Klippel-Trenaunay syndrome. A rare, sporadic, congenital vascular disorder of unknown cause characterized by the triad of overgrowth and hypertrophy of soft tissues and bones (images 1-4), hemangiomas (usually of the port wine type [image 1]), and varicose veins — all on the same side. All three elements, however, are not invariably present and are not necessarily proportionate in severity or extent. These abnormalities may be localized to one extremity or affect as much as an entire half of the body. When the involved tissues contain hemodynamically significant arteriovenous communications, the condition is called the Klippel-Trenaunay-Weber syndrome.

In most cases, the hemangiomas are evident at birth or shortly thereafter, while the soft tissue and bony changes become more apparent after several years. Varicosities are not usually detected until the child spends more time upright.

Associated findings may include digital anomalies, hemangioma-related urinary and rectal bleeding, and various lymphatic disturbances, especially lymphedema (image 5).

Prognosis is good, and treatment is mainly symptomatic.

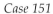

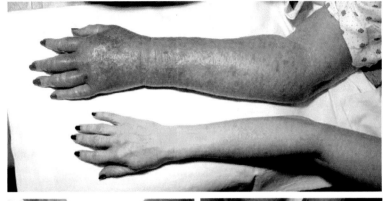

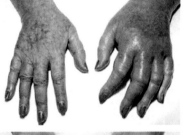

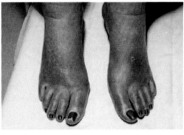

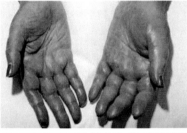

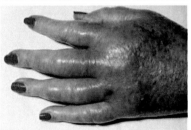

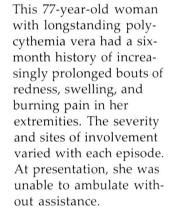

This 77-year-old woman with longstanding polycythemia vera had a six-month history of increasingly prolonged bouts of redness, swelling, and burning pain in her extremities. The severity and sites of involvement varied with each episode. At presentation, she was unable to ambulate without assistance.

151. Erythromelalgia. This rare condition derives its name from the Greek words *erythros* (redness), *melos* (extremity), and *algos* (pain). Swelling and increased skin temperature are its other cardinal features. An alternative term, erythermalgia, emphasizes the warmth and inflammation evident in the affected areas. Although erythromelalgia may appear without underlying disease, it occurs most often with a myelo-proliferative disorder. Sometimes, it precedes the disorder by months to years.

Symptoms frequently begin with an itching sensation followed by burning pain. Fingers, toes, or the entire limb may be affected, and involvement may be unilateral or bilateral, symmetric or asymmetric. The redness and swelling ordinarily resolve within several days, but may, as in the patient shown, last for several weeks. If left untreated, this condition may progress to dystrophic changes, painful acrocyanosis, or peripheral gangrene. Heat, standing, and exercise frequently bring on or aggravate the symptoms while resting, elevating, or cooling the involved limb gives relief.

When erythromelalgia accompanies a myeloproliferative disorder, histologic examination of affected tissue shows fibromuscular and intimal proliferation of the dermal arterioles with narrowing of their lumens. In more advanced cases, thrombi are evident. These lesions are thought to result from platelet activation and aggregation in vivo, with *in situ* thrombosis.

Specific treatment of these patients consists of aspirin to impair platelet aggregation combined with myelosuppressive agents designed to reduce the circulating platelet mass. Such measures in the patient shown afforded substantial clinical improvement.

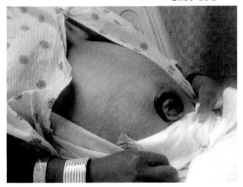

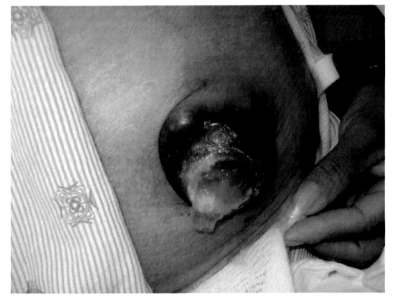

This 38-year-old, healthy-appearing woman presented with increasing abdominal girth of six months' duration and a six-day history of a clear-yellow, gooey substance oozing from her umbilicus.

152. Pseudomyxoma peritonei (PMP). Also known as "jelly belly," PMP is a unique disorder characterized by the accumulation of gelatinous material throughout the abdomen and pelvis together with mucinous implants on the peritoneal surfaces. It is associated with mucin-producing neoplasms—benign and malignant—originating most often in the appendix and ovary. The chief clinical features are conspicuous gelatinous ascites, no visceral invasion or extraperitoneal spread, indolent course, and striking disparity between the extent of disease and the patient's general well-being.

Diagnostic confirmation usually requires laparotomy or laparoscopy, because the pathognomonic peritoneal fluid ordinarily is too thick to aspirate through a needle. Treatment consists primarily of repetitive "debulking surgery." Adjuvant measures include external beam radiotherapy, intraperitoneal radioisotopes, and intraperitoneal or systemic chemotherapy.

The patient shown may be the first with PMP in whom the diagnosis spontaneously "oozed upon the scene." At laparotomy, a yellowish, mucinous material filled her peritoneal cavity (below left) and firmly encased all of her abdominal and pelvic organs (below right). Multiple sections of the peritoneum and umbilicus showed no tumor cells.

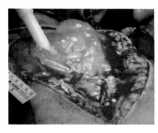

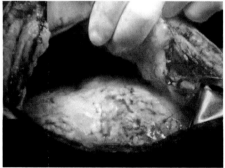

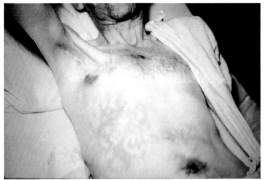

This 63-year-old man sought medical attention for abdominal pain of six months' duration. He also had experienced the recent onset of a gritty yellow discharge from his umbilicus.

Case 154

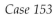

153. Disseminated actinomycosis. On physical examination, this patient had findings that, when taken together, are virtually pathognomonic of actinomycosis: an erythematous, indurated, and tender soft tissue mass in the right paracervical area ("lumpy jaw"); a similar mass in the right axilla; and an indurated, discolored umbilicus with a draining sinus therein. Another draining sinus was evident in the sternum. Cultures of these drainages grew *Actinomyces israelli*. During a year of penicillin therapy, all of the aforementioned abnormalities resolved.

One other point. This patient also had erythema ab igne (arrows, image below), a permanent brown to red, reticulated, residual pigmentation produced by prolonged exposure to excessive nonburning heat. It came about in this man from his use of a heating pad to relieve the abdominal pain.

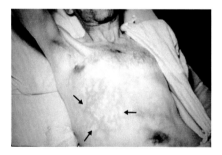

154. Yellow-Nail syndrome. This patient had a 20-year history of severe lymphedema of her legs; thick, ridged, yellowish, hypercurved thumbnails (top right); similarly affected, yellow-green to brown toenails (bottom right); and bilateral, chylous pleural effusions. A sample of her chylous pleural fluid is shown to the left of the radiograph. This syndrome of yellow nails, lymphedema, and pleural effusions (usually serous) presumably results from defective lymphatic drainage. Women are affected almost twice as much as men, and prolonged survival is the rule.

EPILOGUE

In attempting to provide a memorable conclusion, we came across the following thought-provoking quotation:

> *If the only tool you have is a hammer, you tend to see every problem as a nail.*
>
> **Abraham Maslow**

In that light, we hope that this book has helped you find diagnostic tools that you didn't know you had.
If it didn't, . . .

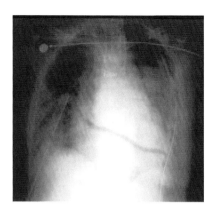

we are heart-broken—like the "broken heart" in the image above.

That heart, by the way, belonged to a 69-year-old woman who had undergone a coronary artery bypass procedure on Valentine's Day. Postoperatively, the portable chest radiograph shown above disclosed a striking radiolucent line bisecting the patient's heart. But on a follow-up radiograph made several hours later, the line had disappeared, proving that it was an artifact and not the result of the surgeon's knife (or Cupid's arrow). The cause of the artifact remains a mystery.

That said, we hope you have enjoyed this journey as much as we have enjoyed charting it.

Original Publication Sources

Some of the images in this book have been published previously in various medical journals and are reprinted here with full permission from those journals. The cases involved and their corresponding publication sources are listed below.

Case	Publication Source
1	Arch Intern Med, 113:866-871 (June) 1964.
2	Practical Gastroenterology, 27:41-42 (March) 2003.
3	Hospital Practice, 34:124-126 (September 1) 1999.
4	Hospital Practice, 29:14 (October 15) 1994.
5	Hospital Practice, 31:148 (May 15) 1996.
6	Practical Gastroenterology, 21:44 (November) 1997.
7	Hospital Practice, 30:24-24p (December 15) 1995.
8	Hospital Practice, 30:102 (January 15) 1995.
9	Hospital Practice, 31:22J (August 15) 1996.
10	Hospital Practice, 30:31 (March 15) 1995.
12	Hospital Practice, 31:123-124 (April 15) 1996.
13	Circulation, 91:3020-3021 (June 15) 1995.
14	Res Staf Phys, 50:26, 34 (December) 2004.
15	Circulation, 107:2870 (June 10) 2003.
16	Hospital Practice, 31:87-91 (December) 1996.
18	Hospital Practice, 32:40 (June 15) 1997.
20	Hospital Practice, 30:24 (June 15) 1995.
21	Hospital Practice, 32:182 (February 15) 1997.
22	Practical Gastroenterology, 26:62, 64 (Nov) 2002.
23	Hospital Practice, 32:24 (July 15) 1997.
24	Res Staf Phys, 50:27 (June) 2004.
25	Hospital Practice, 31:100-102 (September 15) 1996.
26	New Engl J Med, 271:544-546 (September 10) 1964.

Case	Publication Source
27	Hospital Practice, 32:232 (May 15) 1997.
28, 29	Res Staf Phys, 50:45 (November) 2004.
30	Hospital Practice, 30:27 (November 15) 1995.
31	Res Staf Phys, 49:40 (December) 2003.
34	Res Staf Phys, 51:33 (April) 2005.
35	Practical Gastroenterology, 26:50, 52 (October) 2002.
36	Hospital Practice, 32:43-44 (November 15) 1997.
37	Hospital Practice, 31:37-38 (January 15) 1996.
38	Hospital Practice, 29:39 (January15) 1994.
39	Hospital Practice, 33:43 (September 15) 1998.
40, 41, 42	Res Staf Phys, 51:44, (July) 2005.
43	Practical Gastroenterology, 26:46, 48 (July) 2002.
44	Hospital Practice, 34:124-126 (September 1) 1999.
45	New Engl J Med, 340:1969 (June 24) 1999.
46	Circulation, 90:2546 (November) 1994.
47	Hospital Practice, 32:69-70 (April 15) 1997.
49	Hospital Practice, 30:28R-28U (September 15) 1995.
50	Hospital Practice, 31:157-158 (June 15) 1996.
51, 52	Hospital Practice, 33:130 (July 15) 1998.
53	Practical Gastroenterology, 26:72-73 (March) 2002.
55, 56	Hospital Practice, 33:52 (April 15) 1998.
57	Practical Gastroenterology, 26:81-82 (September) 2002.
58, 59, 60	Practical Gastroenterology, 27:41-42 (March) 2003.
61	Hospital Practice, 33:101-107 (December 15) 1998.
62	Hospital Practice, 29:16 (December 15) 1994.
63	Hospital Practice, 34:124-126 (September 1) 1999.
64	Res Staf Phys, 51:26, 36 (July) 2005.
65	Res Staf Phys, 53:43 (May) 2007.

Case	Publication Source
67	Hospital Practice, 34:124-126 (September 1) 1999.
68	Hospital Practice, 31:119-120 (July 15) 1996.
69	Hospital Practice, 29:98 (June 15) 1994.
70	Practical Gastroenterology, 26:36-37 (December) 2002.
71	Res Staf Phys, 50:18, 27 (February) 2004.
72	Hospital Practice, 34:124-126 (September 1) 1999.
74	Hospital Practice, 31:76 (March 15) 1996.
75	Hospital Practice. 31:73-74 (February 15) 1996.
76	Res Staf Phys, 51:26, 36 (July) 2005.
77	Practical Gastroenterology, 26:39, 40, 42 (Oct) 2002.
79	Hospital Practice, 34:124-126 (September 1) 1999.
80	Am Rev Respir Dis, 96:1233-1235 (December) 1967.
82	Am Fam Physician/GP, 1:93 (June) 1970.
92	Am Fam Physician/GP, 1:93 (June) 1970.
95	Practical Gastroenterology, 26:48-49 (January) 2002.
97	GP, 39:92-94 (March) 1969.
100	Practical Gastroenterology, 26:46, 48 (August) 2002.
102	Am J Med, 29:508-517 (September) 1960.
105	South Med J, 85:33-34 (January) 1992.
107	Hospital Practice, 30:66-68 (February 15) 1995.
113	Chest, 57:333-335 (April) 1970.
120	Hospital Practice, 32:182 (February 15) 1997.
143	Hospital Practice, 32:204-208 (May 15) 1997.
148	Hospital Practice, 31:45-49 (November 15) 1996.
150	Res Staf Phys, 52:39 (June) 2006.
154	Res Staf Phys, 50:36 (February) 2004.
Epilogue	Circulation, 105:779 (February 12) 2002.

INDEX

abscess
    breast, 85-86
    liver
        amebic, 87-88
        pyogenic, 63-64
    lung, 85-86, 87-88
    perinephric, 27-28
    tooth, 59-60
achalasia, 99-100
acrocyanosis, 156
acromegaly, 40
acropachy, thyroid, 145-146
acroparesthesias, 74
Actinomyces israelli, 160
actinomycosis
    breast, chest wall, and lungs, 85-86
    disseminated, 159-160
    sternum, 159-160
adenoma sebaceum, 124, 143-144
α-galactosidase A, 74
AIDS, 26, 43-44, 61-62, 67-68
alcaptonuria, 141-142
alopecia, 55-56, 118
amebiasis
    liver, 87-88
    pulmonary, 87-88
ampulla of Vater, 14
amyloidosis, 29-30, 39-40, 72
aneurysms
    dissecting aortic, 33-34, 118
    micro, 23-24
    pulmonary arterial, 117-118
angiitis, hypersensitivity, 126
angiogram, renal, 23-24
angiography, fluorescein, 22
angioid streaks, 57-58
angiokeratomas, 73-74
antiphospholipid-antibody syndrome, 114
aorta, chronic dissection, 33-34, 118
appendix, 158
argyria, 11-12
arteriovenous malformations, 120, 154
arthritis
    reactive, 31-32
    rheumatoid, 50
articular hypermobility, 58

ascites
  gelatinous, 157-158
  myxedema, 89-90, 97-98
  ovarian carcinoma, 15-16
"ash-leaf" macules, 123-124
aspergillosis, sternum, 138
asphyxia, traumatic, 35-36, 107-108
aspirin, 156
atrial septal defect, secundum type, 19-20

Babesia species, 85-86
babesiosis, 85-86
bacteremia, 67-68, 130
bactrim, 114
balanitis circinata, 31-32
bartonellosis, 144
"bathing suit" area, 74
blood film, peripheral
  Babesia species, 85-86
  basophilic stippling, 87-88
  Borrelia hermsii, 9-10
  Ehrlichia phagocytophilia, 51-52
  Histoplasma capsulatum, 25-26
  Loa loa, 71-72
  Streptococcus pneumoniae, 67-68
  Trypanosoma cruzi, 77-78
blue rubber-bleb nevus syndrome, 45-46
bones, fragile, 50
Borrelia hermsii, 9-10
botulism, wound, 47-48
Bournville disease, 124
Branham's sign, 132
breast
  actinomycosis, 85-86
  eyelid metastases, 81-82
  infiltrating lobular carcinoma, 81-82
bronchogenic carcinoma, 19-20, 33-34, 41-42, 67-68, 129-130, 147-148
"bronzed diabetes," 149-150
brucellosis, sternum, 138
Bruch's membrane, 58

café-au-lait spots, 95-96, 116
Calabar swellings, 72
calcific retinal emboli, 13-14
calcification
  gallbladder wall, 27-28
  intervertebral discs, 142

pancreas, 51-52
pericardium, 53-54
Candida species, 12
carcinoid syndrome, 127-128
carcinoma
    ampulla of Vater, 14
    breast, 81-82
    bronchogenic, 19-20, 33-34, 41-42, 67-68, 129-130, 147-148
    gallbladder, 28
    kidney, 83-84, 137-138
    neck, 131-132
    ovary, 15-16, 93-94
    pancreas, 37-38, 93-94, 137-138
    penile, 148
    prostate, 81-82
    stomach, 93-94
    thyroid, 84, 121-122
cataracts, 117-118
catheter, central venous, 151-152
Chagas disease, 77-78
chancre, syphilitic, 62, 147-148
chancroid, 148
"charcoal heart," 149-150
chemotherapy, 82, 84, 116, 158
chills, 27, 63, 67, 95-96, 105
Chlamydia trachomatis, 18
clofazimine, 114
clostridia, 12
Clostridium botulinum, 48
clubbing, 133-134, 146
cocaine, 125-126
coccidioidomycosis, sternum, 138
colon interposition, 77-78
complement system, 68
computed tomography, 28, 34, 54, 60, 64, 76, 111, 131-132
conjunctivae
    comma-shaped or cork-screw-shaped vessels, 35-36
    hemorrhage, 35-36, 105-106, 107-108
    lymphoma, 69-70, 83-84
    petechiae, 95-96
    Romaña's sign, 78
Contarini's condition, 109-110
coumarin, 91-92
cranial nerve palsies, 25-26, 47-48, 99-100, 111-112
Crohn's disease, 72
cryoglobulinemia, 135-136
crystals, sodium urate, 40
culdocentesis, 15-16
Cullen's sign, 123-124

Cushing's disease, 99-100
cyclophosphamide, 82
cyclosporine, 72
cystic medial necrosis, 117-118
cystitis emphysematosa, 11-12
cytomegalovirus, 72

dapsone, 114
deafness, 50
death, 64
"debulking surgery," 158
dementia, 64
dental sinus tract, 59-60
dermatitis, 64
dermatomyositis, 41-42
Descemet's membrane, 18
diarrhea, 45, 64, 127
diltiazem, 72
diplococci, 67-68
discs, calcified intervertebral, 142
disease
     Addison's, 100
     Bournville, 124
     Chagas, 77-78
     Crohn's, 72
     Cushing's, 99-100
     Fabry's, 73-74
     Fong's, 101-102
     Graves', 103-104
     Hansen's, 107-108
     Hodgkin's, 137-138
     Marfan's, 50
     Milroy's, 15
     Osler-Weber-Rendu, 119-120
     Wilson's, 17-18
disorder, myeloproliferative, 156
drug reactions, 114
dysphagia, 99
dyssebacia, 63-64

Ebstein's anomaly, 91
ecchymoses, 31-32, 75-76, 123-124
Ehlers – Danlos syndrome, 50, 57-58
Ehrlichia phagocytophilia, 51-52
ehrlichiosis, human granulocytic, 51-52
elbows, 101-102

emboli
    fat, 95-96
    mercury, 21-22
    retinal, calcific, 13-14
eosinophilic pneumonia, 37-38
eosinophils, 38
epiloia, 124
epistaxis, 125
erythema ab igne, 159-160
erythermalgia, 156
erythromelalgia, 155-156
Escherichia coli, 12
esophagus, 99-100
exophthalmos, 25-26, 97-98, 103-104, 145-146
eyebrows, 21-22, 107-108
eyelashes, 21-22, 107-108
eyelids
    hemorrhage, 29-30
    metastases, 81-82
    swollen, 83, 103
    thickening and induration, 81-82
    waxy papules, 29-30, 139-140
eyes
    blue sclerae, 49-50, 142
    false, 37-38
    Kayser-Fleischer ring, 17-18
    lipemia retinalis, 53-54
    melanoma, 37-38
    "raccoon," 29-30
    subcapsular lenticular opacity, 104

Fabry's disease, 73-74
face
    adenoma sebaceum, 143-144
    discoloration, blue-red to blue-black, 35-36, 107-108
    leprosy, 107-108
    malignant syphilis, 143-144
    neurofibromatosis Type 2, 115-116
fibromas
    gingival, 72, 124
    periungual, 124
fistula
    arteriovenous, 131-132
    tracheoesophageal, 78
fluorescein angiography, 22
5-fluorouracil, 82
flushing, 127-128

Fong's disease, 101-102
Foramen of Morgagni hernia, 59-60
Fox's sign, 31-32
Francisella tularensis, 114
freckling, 96

gallbladder
    carcinoma, 28
    porcelain, 27-28
gangrene
    jejunum, 47-48
    peripheral, 135-136, 156
    symmetric peripheral, 23-24
gas
    biliary tract, 48
    portal vein, 47-48
    urinary bladder wall, 11-12
glioma, 104
glioma, optic nerve, 96
glycosphingolipids, 74
gonadal atrophy, 118
gonococcal dermatitis, 129-130
Gottron's papules, 41-42
gout, tophaceous, 39-40
granuloma inguinale, 148
Graves' disease, 103-104
groove sign, 17-18
gumma, 111-112
gums
    acute myelomonocytic leukemia, 71-72
    fibromas, 124
    hypertrophy (differential diagnosis), 72
    keratosis, 7-8
    lymphoma, 72
    scurvy, 75-76

hamartomas, iris, 96
Hansen's disease, 107-108
Heart
    atrial septal defect, 19-20
    block, 117
    "broken," 162
    "charcoal," 149-150
    Ebstein's anomaly, 91
    metastases, 149-150
    tetralogy of Fallot, 133-134

hemangiomas
  cutaneous, 153-154
  visceral, 46
hematemesis, 57
hemihypertrophy, bones and soft tissues, 153-154
hemochromatosis, 149-150
hemorrhages, perifollicular, 75-76
hepatolenticular degeneration, 18
hereditary gingival fibromatosis, 72
hereditary hemorrhagic telangiectasia, 119-120
hereditary osteo-onycho-dysplasia (HOOD), 101-102
hernia, Foramen of Morgagni, 59-60
Histoplasma capsulatum, 26
histoplasmosis, disseminated, 25-26
Hodgkin's disease, sternum, 137-138
Hoffman's syndrome, 121-122
homogentisic acid oxidase, 142
HOOD, 101-102
hyperbilirubinemia, 37-38
hyperkeratosis, 7-8
hypersensitivity angiitis, 126
hyperthyroidism, 97-98, 145-146
hypogammaglobulinemia, 68
hyposplenism, 68
hypothyroidism, 40, 89-90, 97-98, 121-122

iliac horns, 101-102
inflammatory bowel disease, 114
interferon, 116
intimal flap, 34
iris hamartomas, 96
iron
  deficiency, 50
  excess, 150

"jelly belly," 157-158
joints, hypermobile, 58

Kaposi's sarcoma, 72
Kayser-Fleischer ring, 17-18
keratosis
  gums, 7-8
  keratoderma blenorrhagica, 44
  palmaris et plantaris, 7-8
  pellagrous, 9-10

psoriatic, 43-44
seborrheic, 15-16,129-130
tongue, 7-8
Klebsiella pneumoniae, 64
Klebsiella rhinoscleromatis, 62
Klippel-Trenaunay syndrome, 153-154
Klippel-Trenaunay-Weber syndrome, 154

laparoscopy, 158
laparotomy, 158
larvae
    gut, 45-46
    urine, 45-46
lead poisoning, 87-88
Leishmania brasiliensis, 114
leishmaniasis, 144
lens, opacity, 104, 118
leprosy, 107-108, 112, 144
Leptospira icterohemorrhagiae, 105-106
leptospirosis, 105-106
Leser-Trélat sign, 15-16,129-130
lethal midline granuloma, 125-126
leukemia, acute myelomonocytic, 71-72
l'homme rouge, 116
lipemia retinalis, 53-54
lipogranuloma, 105-106
liposarcoma, 75-76
lips
    hemorrhage, 29-30
    neuromas, 121-122
    telangiectases, 119-120
Lisch nodules, 96
Loa loa, 71-72
loiasis, 71-72
"lumpy jaw," 159-160
lymphangitis, nodular, 114
lymphedema, 153-154, 159-160
lymphogranuloma venereum, 17-18, 148
lymphoma
    conjunctival, 69-70, 83-84
    cutaneous, 115-116
    gums, 72
    inguinal (simulating infection), 55-56
lymphomatoid granulomatosis, 111-112

malaria, *Plasmodium falciparum*, 86
Marfan's disease, 50

melanoma, metastatic, 89-90, 149-150
membrane, Bruch's, 53
meningioma, 104
meningitis, aseptic, 22
meningococcemia, 96
mercury emboli, 21-22
metastases
    cutaneous, 15-16, 33-34, 41-42
    eyelids, 81-82
    osteoblastic, 81-82
    osteolytic, 82, 84
    pulmonary, 89-90
    pulsatile, 83-84, 137-138
    umbilical, 93-94
methotrexate, 82
microfilariae, 71-72
"midline granuloma" syndrome, 125-126
Milroy's disease, 15
minocycline, 114
mitral annulus, calcified, 14
morula, 51-52
mucormycosis, rhinocerebral, 25-26
multiple endocrine neoplasia (MEN-II B), 121-122
multiple myeloma, 69-70, 135-136, 137-138
myasthenia gravis, 50, 109-110
Mycobacterium leprae, 108
Mycobacterium marinum, 114
mycosis fungoides, 44, 144
myeloproliferative disorder, 156
myopathy, hypothyroid, 121-122
myotonic dystrophy, 117-118
myxedema
    ascites, 89-90, 97-98
    pretibial, 145-146

nail-patella syndrome, 101-102
nails
    dysplastic, 101-102
    yellow, 159-160
necrosis
    cheek, ear, and feet, 135-136
    fingers and toes, 23-24
    nose and palate, 25-26
    pulpal, 60
    thigh, 91-92
neck
    AV fistula, 131-132
    squamous cell carcinoma, 131-132

Nelson's syndrome, 99-100
nephrotic syndrome, 20
neurofibromatosis
    Type 1, 95-96, 133-134
    Type 2, 103-104, 115-116
neuromas
    lips, 121-122
    tongue, 121-122
niacin, 10
nifedipine, 72
Nocardia brasiliensis, 114
Nocardia species, 12
nodules, Lisch, 96
nose
    mass, 61-62
    septal perforation, 125-126

ochronosis, 141-142
ophthalmoplegia
    external, 25-26, 99-100
    total, 47-48
optic nerve glioma, 96
oropharynx, 61-62
Osler-Weber-Rendu disease, 119-120
osteogenesis imperfecta, 49-50
ovary, 158
ovary, carcinoma, 15-16, 93-94

palate
    hard, 25-26
    soft, 125-126
pancreas
    calcification, 51-52
    carcinoma, 37-38, 93-94, 137-138
pancreatitis, acute, 31-32, 123-124
paracentesis, 15-16, 158
patella, 42, 101-102
pellagra, 9-10, 63-64
penicillamine, 72
penile carcinoma, 148
penis, 31
peritoneum, 158
petechiae, 95-96
phenol compounds, 142
phenytoin, 72
pheochromocytoma, 122
photophobia, 81

photophoresis, 116
pituitary, 100
plasmacytomas, 69-70, 137-138
plasmapheresis, 146
Plasmodium falciparum, 86
platelet, 156
pleural effusions
    bloody, 109-110
    chylous, 109-110, 159-160
pneumomediastinum, 127-128
pneumonia, eosinophilic, 37-38
poliosis, 21-22
polyarteritis nodosa, 23-24
polycythemia vera, 155
prognathism, 122
prostate, metastatic carcinoma, 81-82
Proteus mirabilis, 28
pruritus, 61-62, 79-80, 115-116
pseudomyxoma peritonei, 157-158
pseudoxanthoma elasticum, 50, 57-58
psoriasiform lesions, 61-62, 65, 79
psoriasis, 43-44
ptosis, 25-26, 47-48, 99-100, 109-110
pulmonary arterial aneurysm, 117-118
pulmonic stenosis, 128
pulpal necrosis, 60
pulsatile scrotal mass, 91-92
pyoderma gangrenosum, 113-114, 144

quinacrine, 142
quinones, 142

radiotherapy, 70, 84, 98, 100, 104, 116, 126, 158
Reiter's syndrome, 31-32
relapsing fever, 9-10
renal cell carcinoma, 83-84, 137-138
retina
    angioid streaks, 57-58
    calcific emboli, 13-14
    detachment, 22
    leaks, 22
    lipemia, 53-54
rheumatoid arthritis, 50
rhinoscleroma, 61-62
ribs
    multiple myeloma, 69-70
    prostatic carcinoma, 81-82

"ring around the artery" sign, 127-128
Romaña's sign, 77-78
rouleaux formation, 135

sarcoidosis
    bony, 139-140
    cutaneous, 65-66, 139-140
    dactylitis, 139-140
    gums, 72
    phalangeal, 139-140
Sarcoptes scabiei, 79-80
scabies, 79-80
scabies, Norwegian, 44
Schwannoma, 104
sclerae
    blue, 49-50, 142
    brown-black spot, 142
    icteric, 37-38, 105-106
scrotum
    pulsating mass (causes), 92
    varices, 91-92
scurvy
    ecchymoses, 75-76
    gums, 72, 75-76
    perifollicular hemorrhages, 75-76
sebum, inspissated, 64
Sézary cells, 115-116
Sézary syndrome, 115-116
shagreen patches, 124
shoulder pad sign, 39-40
sickle cell disease, 35-36
sign
    Branham's, 132
    conjunctival, 35-36
    Cullen's, 123-124
    Fox's, 31-32
    groove, 17-18
    Leser-Trélat, 15-16, 129-130
    "ring around the artery," 127-128
    Romaña's, 77-78
    shoulder pad, 39-40
    Turner's, 31-32
silver
    nose drops, 11-12
    stool, 13-14
sinuses
    actinomycotic, 85-86, 157-158
    dental, 59-60

skin
    angiokeratomas, 73-74
    "ash-leaf" macules, 123-124
    blue, 11-12, 141-142
    bullae, 91-92, 129-130, 135-136
    "cigarette paper," 58
    desquamation, 10
    ecchymoses, 31-32, 75-76, 123-124
    erythema ab igne, 157-158
    erythema and scaling, 10, 41-42
    fibromas
        gingival, 124
        periungual, 124
    flushing, 127-128
    hemangiomas, 153-154
    hemorrhagic, 129-130
    hyperelastic, 57-58
    hyperpigmentation, 99-100, 149-150
    ichthyosis, 65-66
    keratosis, 7-8, 9-10, 15-16, 43-44, 129-130
    livedo reticularis, 135-136
    metastases, 15-16, 33-34, 41-42
    necrosis, 23-24, 91-92, 129-130, 135-136
    nodules, 61-62, 65-66, 82, 83-84, 107-108
    papules, 61-62, 65-66, 73-74, 79-80, 111-112, 139-140
    papulopustular, 143-144
    petechiae, 95-96
    plaques, 43-44, 65-66, 107-108
    "plucked chicken," 57-58
    pruritus, 61-62, 79-80, 115-116
    shagreen patches, 124
    spiders, 119-120
    telangiectases, 119-120, 127-128
    ulcerative, 113-114
    vascular malformations, 45-46
    venous stars, 67-68, 147-148
    vesiculopustular, 129-130
    vitiligo, 21-22
"soap-bubble" syndrome, 105-106
spider bites, 114
spiders, giant arterial, 119-120
spine, 142
spirochetes, 9-10, 62, 144, 148
Sporothrix schencki, 114
sporotrichosis, 113-114
squamous cell carcinoma, 41-42, 67-68, 129-130, 131-132
staphylococci, 12

sternum
    actinomycosis, 159-160
    aspergillosis, 138
    brucellosis, 138
    coccidioidomycosis, 138
    Hodgkin's disease, 137-138
    multiple myeloma, 137-138
    pancreatic carcinoma, 137-138
    pseudomonal disease, 138
    renal cell carcinoma, 137-138
    staphylococcal disease, 138
    tuberculosis, 138
stippling of red cells, 87-88
stomach, carcinoma, 93-94
stool
    black, 57
    silver, 13-14
Streptococcus pneumoniae, 67-68
Strongyloides stercoralis, 45-46
strongyloidiasis, disseminated, 45-46
sulfur granules, 86
superior vena caval syndrome, 147-148
syndrome
    antiphospholipid-antibody, 114
    blue rubber-bleb nevus, 45-46
    carcinoid, 127-128
    Ehlers – Danlos, 57-58
    Hoffman's, 121-122
    Klippel-Trenaunay, 153-154
    Klippel-Trenaunay-Weber, 154
    "midline granuloma," 125-126
    nail-patella, 101-102
    Nelson's, 99-100
    nephrotic, 20
    Reiter's, 31-32
    Sézary, 115-116
    "soap-bubble," 105-106
    superior vena caval, 147-148
    Vogt-Koyanagi-Harada, 21-22
    yellow-nail, 157-158
syphilis
    cerebral gumma, 111-112
    chancre, 62, 147-148
    malignant, 143-144
    secondary, 61-62

tearing, excessive, 81, 104

teeth
 abscess, 59-60
 blue, 141-142
 root disease, 59-60
telangiectases, 119-120, 127-128
Tensilon, 109-110
tetralogy of Fallot, 133-134
thallium, acute poisoning, 55-56
thyroid
 acropachy, 145-146
 carcinoma, 84, 121-122
 hyper, 97-98, 145-146
 hypo, 89-90, 97-98, 121-122
 thyromegaly, 146
tongue
 keratosis, 7-8
 neuromas, 121-122
 serrated, 39-40
 telangiectases, 119-120
tophi, 39-40
traumatic asphyxia, 35-36, 107-108
Treponema pallidum, 147-148
tricuspid insufficiency, 92
triglycerides, serum, 54
Trypanosoma cruzi, 77-78
trypanosomiasis, 77-78
trypomastigote, 77-78
tuberculosis, sternum, 138
tuberous sclerosis, 123-124, 143-144
tumor, cranial nerve VIII, 104
Turner's sign, 31-32

ulnar palsies, 111-112
umbilical metastases, 93-94
umbilicus, 123-124, 157-158, 159-160
urine, black, 142
uveitis, 22

varicocele, pulsating, 91-92
vasculitis, 114
veins
 collaterals, 15-16, 49-50
 portal, 47-48
 varicose, 91-92, 153-154
vena cava, inferior
 obstruction, 15-16, 49-50

vena cava, superior
    obstruction, bronchogenic carcinoma, 19-20, 147-148
venous stars, 67-68, 147-148
verapamil, 72
vitiligo, 21-22
Vogt-Koyanagi-Harada syndrome, 21-22

Wegener's granulomatosis, 72, 112, 126
Wilson's disease, 17-18

yaws, 144
yellow-nail syndrome, 159-160

ABOUT THE AUTHORS

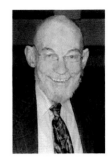

Herbert L. Fred, MD, MACP, is one of the nation's best-known medical educators and diagnosticians. He is the author of more than 400 publications, including three books—each a collection of provocative essays—providing philosophical insights into disease, the practice of medicine, the challenge of difficult diagnoses, the joys, frustrations, and rewards of teaching, the pleasurable pain of learning, and the exhilaration of true scholarship. Among his many awards is a Presidential Citation, given him by President Ronald Reagan in 1988. The American College of Physicians named him its Distinguished Teacher for 2004, and awarded him Mastership the same year. In 2005, he received the TIAA-CREF Distinguished Medical Educator Award. The Herb Fred Medical Society, Inc., founded in 2002 by Dr. Fred's former trainees, honors him for "a half century of bedside teaching." Dr. Fred is an emeritus member of the American Osler Society and has served on the editorial boards of numerous national medical journals. He is currently Professor of Medicine at The University of Texas Health Science Center at Houston. He lives in Houston with his wife, Judy. They have seven children.

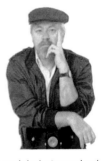

For more than 40 years, Hendrik A. van Dijk has authored, produced or directed audio-visual projects, educational films and videos, still photographs, book illustrations, and slide presentations about medicine. After his training as an aerial photographer/cartographer by the Dutch Royal Air Force and his subsequent graduation from the Dutch School for Professional Photography in The Hague, Mr. van Dijk made his way to Duke University in 1968, where he began working in biomedical communications. He has gone on to become one of the nation's leading experts in that field. Most recently, he was Director of the Graphic Communications Group at the University of Texas Health Science Center at Houston, until his retirement in 2005. He lives in Houston, Texas, with his wife Yoka. They have two children.